JEN HOBBS

COOKING
with
CBD

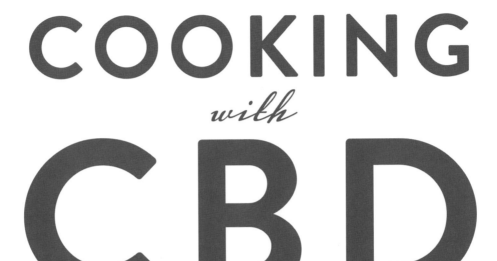

50 DELICIOUS CANNABIDIOL- AND HEMP-INFUSED RECIPES FOR WHOLE-BODY HEALING WITHOUT THE HIGH

ULYSSES PRESS

For my daughter—the pickiest eater I know—who'll always be my source of laughter and inspiration, and who's now learned a thing or two about mixing eggs and inventing recipes of her own.

Published in the U.S. by:
Ulysses Press
P.O. Box 3440
Berkeley, CA 94703
www.ulyssespress.com

ISBN: 978-1-64604-035-3
Library of Congress Control Number: 2020931880

Printed in the United States by Versa Printing
10 9 8 7 6 5 4 3 2 1

Acquisitions editor: Claire Sielaff
Project editor: Tyanni Niles
Managing editor: Claire Chun
Editor: Phyllis Elving
Proofreader: Renee Rutledge
Cover design: Rebecca Lown
Interior design and layout: what!design @ whatweb.com
Photographs: © Jen Hobbs except pages 5 and 128 © Rocio Martinez/Rocio Beauty Pixels

NOTE TO READERS: This book has been written and published strictly for informational and educational purposes only. It is not intended to serve as medical advice or to be any form of medical treatment. You should always consult your physician before altering or changing any aspect of your medical treatment and/or undertaking a diet regimen, including the guidelines as described in this book. Do not stop or change any prescription medications without the guidance and advice of your physician. Any use of the information in this book is made on the reader's good judgment after consulting with his or her physician and is the reader's sole responsibility. This book is not intended to diagnose or treat any medical condition and is not a substitute for a physician. The author and publisher disclaim liability for any medical outcomes that may occur as a result of applying the methods suggested in this book.

This book is independently authored and published and no sponsorship or endorsement of this book by, and no affiliation with, any trademarked brands or other products mentioned within is claimed or suggested. All trademarks that appear in ingredient lists and elsewhere in this book belong to their respective owners and are used here for informational purposes only. The author and publisher encourage readers to patronize the quality brands mentioned in this book.

CONTENTS

INTRODUCTION

Cooking with CBD is a collection of meals that I enjoy making. I developed many of these recipes when my husband and I were growing medical marijuana in California, and revising them for this cookbook brought back such fond memories. Today, living in a suburb of St. Louis, we are far removed from those days of raising free-range chickens, waking up to the annoyingly inconsistent call of our rooster (his internal clock was completely off), and having an endless supply of fruit because crisp green apples, juicy red grapes, sugary figs, and wild blackberries grew all over the property.

Of course, cooking with CBD—cannabidiol—isn't the same as cooking with marijuana. None of the recipes in this book will get you high because CBD is for people who want to feel better *without* the high. Unless you choose to add THC, the only effect you'll feel is relief from whatever is ailing you.

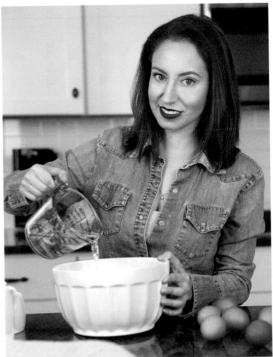

The majority of these recipes take 30 minutes or less to prepare, start to finish. They can be whipped up with minimal planning and without a long list of ingredients. And since every recipe contains CBD, every bite of every meal is sure to melt away anxiety, ease stress, and provide relief for medical conditions.

It's often said that the joy of cooking and baking is in making food for those we love, and through that daily routine we also make a lifetime of family memories. We gather in the kitchen to help or to learn or to enjoy each other's company, and then we talk and share and laugh when we gather around the table to eat. I hope that you enjoy making the recipes in this book and that you're able to create many beautiful memories in the process.

With peace and love,

Jen

Chapter 1
LEARN THE BASICS

In 2013, CNN Chief Medical Correspondent Dr. Sanjay Gupta wrote an op-ed piece titled "Why I Changed My Mind on Weed," in which he apologized for not having considered marijuana to be a medication. "We have been terribly and systematically misled for nearly 70 years in the United States, and I apologize for my own role in that,"[1] he said. This is the same neurosurgeon who had penned the article "Why I Would Vote No on Pot" for *TIME Magazine* in 2009.

He discovered that he'd been misled, Gupta explained, while he was compiling footage for his documentary series *Weed*. He began reading scientific studies published in scholarly medical journals, all of which contradicted the Drug Enforcement Agency's claim that cannabis is one of the most dangerous drugs on the planet, with no accepted medical use. He also spoke with doctors and patients who bore witness to the near-miraculous healing power of medical marijuana.

In September 2019, Gupta's fifth documentary on cannabis (*Weed* 5) aired on CNN, and he commemorated the occasion with another opinion piece—"Dr. Sanjay Gupta on Medical Marijuana: We Are in an Age of Wisdom, but Also an Age of Foolishness." Gupta stated: "Make no mistake: Cannabis is a medicine. . . . At times, it can heal when nothing else can. Denying people this substance represents a moral issue just as much as a medical one."[2]

Gupta cited the case of Charlotte Figi, who had suffered from frequent seizures since she was three months old, lasting two to five hours. At age two and a half she was diagnosed with Dravet syndrome, a rare seizure disorder. By the time she was five, Charlotte could no longer walk or talk and couldn't even eat because of her seizures. She was having 300 grand mal seizures a week, and they were causing her heart to stop.

---

1 Sanjay Gupta, "Why I Changed My Mind on Weed," CNN.com, https://www.cnn.com/2013/08/08/health/gupta-changed-mind-marijuana/index.html (accessed 10/2/19).
2 Sanjay Gupta, "Dr. Sanjay Gupta on Medical Marijuana: We Are in an Age of Wisdom, but Also an Age of Foolishness," CNN.com, https://www.cnn.com/2019/09/27/health/weed-5-cbd-craze-gupta/index.html (accessed 10/2/19).

Doctors didn't expect Charlotte to live past her eighth birthday. There was nothing left to do—except to turn to the one medication no doctor at the time considered prescribing for a child: cannabis. Charlotte's parents had heard about CBD-dominant cannabis strains that were effective in treating Dravet syndrome. Eventually the Figis found a doctor in Colorado who granted Charlotte access to medical marijuana. As a five-year-old, she became the state's youngest medical marijuana patient.

The results were essentially instant; after her mother administered a few drops of cannabis oil on Charlotte's tongue, Charlotte was seizure-free for an hour...and then the next hour...and then the following *seven days*.[3] By age six she was thriving: walking, riding a bicycle, feeding herself, talking. On average she experienced only two or three seizures a month, despite being off all pharmaceutical seizure medications. She took CBD oil twice a day in her food. That's all she needed.

In April 2020, Charlotte Figi passed away at the age of 13 from pneumonia, a likely case of COVID-19, although she tested negative for the virus. Charlotte undeniably lived a better life, thanks to cannabis, and she was an inspiration for many involved in the CBD movement. The CBD oil that Charlotte put in her food is called Charlotte's Web. Derived from hemp, it's non-psychoactive and has a high content of CBD with an extremely low content of THC. Today, Charlotte's Web is just one of many cannabis strains available in CBD oil, lotions, capsules, gummies, and even dog treats. Along with epileptic conditions, CBD has been found to treat many other ailments for which there are limited pharmaceutical options.

COOKING WITH CBD

While taking CBD oil under the tongue is certainly effective, most people find the bitter taste extremely unpleasant. Fortunately, that taste can be masked entirely by adding the oil to food or beverages—

---

3 Saundra Young, "Marijuana Stops Child's Severe Seizures," CNN.com. https://www.cnn.com/2013/08/07/health/charlotte-child-medical-marijuana/index.html (accessed 10/2/19).

which is what this book is all about. In the following pages you'll find all sorts of delicious options for adding CBD to your meals.

For anyone wondering *why go through the trouble* of infusing CBD into food when you can simply smoke or vape it for immediate relief:

1. Taking CBD in food increases its bioavailability. Compared to smoking or vaping, taking CBD in or with food offers a more stable, consistent daily dosing schedule. According to a study published in 2018, CBD's absorption rate increases when it is "administered with food" or when a meal is eaten right after the CBD is consumed. The study concluded that food is required for "optimal absorption" of CBD.[4]

2. Infusing CBD in food is discreet. You can't smoke or vape everywhere, but you can snack on CBD edibles practically anywhere.

3. Eating CBD doesn't harm the lungs. If you have a cough, cold, sinus infection, or medical condition that doesn't allow you to smoke at all, or if your lungs are highly sensitive to smoke, then smoking your medication isn't really an option. But we all have to eat and drink, and adding CBD to foods and beverages won't irritate the lungs.

4. It's effective longer. While smoking CBD can give immediate relief, the effect can fade within an hour. When taken with food, however, the medication stays in your body much longer. You might be able to skip smoking altogether once you figure out the best times of the day to include CBD in your food.

5. You have more control over dosages. If you know your CBD-infused snack will give you three hours of relief, you can plan your day better. Plus, having your medication in your food can minimize the stress of keeping track of how much CBD oil you have on hand.

6. You might save money! Since the medication lasts much longer when it's ingested than when it's vaped or smoked, you may not need to purchase it as much or as often.

WHICH TYPE IS BEST FOR COOKING?

CBD is extracted from the bud, or flower, of the hemp plant—similar to the way lavender and vanilla are extracted from plants. It can be purchased as CBD isolate, broad-spectrum CBD, or full-spectrum CBD, depending on how the CBD was extracted and what kind of cannabinoids are in it (see CBD 101: Your Cannabidiol Reference Guide, page 119). All three types are available as water-soluble CBD—in powder form or, more typically, as a liquid. You can also purchase CBD flower to smoke or infuse into cooking oil or butter.

---

4 Sophie A. Millar, Nicole L. Stone, Andrew S. Yates, Saoirse E. O'Sullivan, "A Systematic Review on the Pharmacokinetics of Cannabidiol in Humans," *Frontiers in Pharmacology* 9 (2018): 1365. https://www.ncbi.nlm.nih.gov/pmc/articles/PMC6275223.

Research indicates that CBD bioavailability increases if it's eaten with food that has a high fat content. Infusing CBD oil with a fat substance such as butter, milk, or cream allows it to bind with the fat, which increases its absorption rate in the body. This is why most people add CBD to butter or cooking oil. When I'm cooking something that doesn't contain a fatty substance, I prefer to use water-soluble CBD in its liquid form because the CBD mixes much more thoroughly with the rest of the ingredients.

The benefit of cooking with water-soluble CBD is that it mixes much more thoroughly with non-fatty substances compared to CBD oil. Think about olive oil and balsamic vinegar salad dressing. You can mix it and shake it, but the oil and vinegar always separate. It's the same with CBD oil that isn't water soluble. If you put CBD oil in coffee, you'll notice little oil droplets on the surface. No matter how much you stir, the CBD oil will separate from the coffee. However, water-soluble CBD goes through a process to decrease the size of the oil particles on the molecular level. The oil particles are so small that water-soluble CBD will "mix" into any liquid (including water) or any food product. Since the human body is about 60 percent water, manufacturers claim water-soluble CBD is up to 10 times more bioavailable than regular CBD oil, meaning you absorb more of it and it works faster. I find water-soluble CBD is particularly useful for beverages, salad dressings, and sauces. Keep in mind that the time it takes for CBD to take effect varies, depending on how it is consumed. When cannabis is smoked or vaped, the effects are nearly immediate but can wear off in about an hour. When CBD oil is infused into edibles, it can take up to 60 minutes for it to start working, but the medication can last anywhere from two to six hours depending on the concentration.

MASKING THE TASTE OF CBD

You might notice these ingredients throughout this book:

- Ginger
- Herbs such as basil, mint, chives
- Garlic
- Peanut butter
- Dark chocolate

- Fruits such as lemon, lime, strawberry, cranberry
- Spice-rack essentials such as cumin, dry mustard, chili powder
- Tart or crisp flavors such as vinegar (apple cider, balsamic) and blue cheese

If you're considering adding CBD to one of your own recipes, keep these flavors in mind, as they work well to mask the bitter taste of CBD. No matter what you're making, from guacamole to chocolate mousse to soup, be sure to stir thoroughly—more than you normally would. This will ensure that the CBD is evenly distributed, giving equal potency to every bite.

You can buy hemp seeds, hemp protein powder, hemp seed cooking oil, hemp milk, and even hemp butter at grocery stores or online. Hemp seeds are considered a superfood because of their incredible nutritional benefits. The seed's plant-based protein is actually a complete protein, offering every single amino acid the human body needs to survive. There are approximately 10 grams of protein and 3 grams of fiber in just 3 tablespoons of hulled hemp seeds, so sprinkling even a small amount on a meal goes a long way.

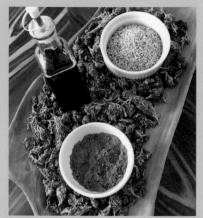

You can cook with hemp protein powder, hemp seeds, hemp seed oil, and hemp flower, but only hemp flower contains CBD.

HEMP SEED can be purchased in two forms—with the shells and without them. Both are edible and delicious, but they differ in texture. Whole (unhulled) hemp seeds means *with* the shell; they are crunchy, and the shell is an excellent source of fiber. Hulled (shelled) hemp seeds are much easier to chew. They're also known as "hemp hearts."

HEMP PROTEIN POWDER is the by-product of hemp seed oil that is milled into a fine, flour-like consistency. A 4-tablespoon serving has 7 to 13 grams of fiber, 13 grams of protein, 2.5 grams of omega-3 and -6, and potassium, magnesium, iron, and calcium. Unlike hemp seeds, the protein powder doesn't have much taste, so it's easily incorporated into smoothies and baked goods.

HEMP SEED OIL is a natural source of essential fatty acids. Cold pressed from hemp seed, this raw, organic, unrefined oil has a strong, nutty taste. It's a phenomenal source of balanced omega-3 and -6. Do not use for frying or heating above 350°F, as the omegas can burn off at high temperatures. Once opened, hemp seed oil needs to be refrigerated, so I use it mainly for recipes that require refrigeration or are meant to be consumed cold, such as smoothies.

MAKING YOUR OWN CBD BUTTER AND COOKING OIL

When I was a kid, Choose Your Own Adventure books were extremely popular. These books let the reader choose what the novel's protagonist would do next. Since there are many ways to infuse CBD into foods and drinks, I'd like you to think of this book as a Choose Your Own Adventure cookbook. If a recipe calls for CBD butter and you don't have any, there are ways to swap it out with regular butter and use CBD cooking oil or water-soluble CBD instead.

If you've cooked or baked with marijuana, the amount you used was likely *way more* than the amount you'll use to cook with CBD. While you can't overdose on CBD, it can be expensive, and we definitely don't want to waste any by going overboard on the dosage.

First and foremost, if you're looking to make your own CBD butter or oil, use a scale so you can accurately weigh the hemp flower in grams and ounces. And regardless of how much CBD you choose to infuse into butter or oil, label each batch with the date and quantity of CBD. This will help you keep track of what you've made so that you can dose up or down, depending on what you're preparing. You might choose to make butter and oil at different strengths for different kinds of recipes, and you don't want to mix up those batches!

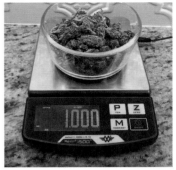

While it may seem like an extra step to make your own cooking oil or butter when these products can be purchased with CBD already in them, I find the main benefit is that I get to choose the strength of the hemp flower and the brand of butter and oil. This means my CBD oil and CBD butter can be *stronger* in potency than store-bought, and I can go with my favorite cooking oils to ensure that I'm using something that's high-quality and organic. If you're wondering how much hemp flower to use for your infusion, see CBD Dosage Calculators on page 123.

WASHING AND DECARBING YOUR HEMP FLOWER. Before infusing CBD into butter or oil, the hemp flower has to go through a decarboxylation process to "activate" the CBD, or convert CBD-A to CBD. But even *before* decarbing the hemp flower, it's a good idea to put it through a rinsing process.

We wash herbs, fruits, and vegetables before eating or cooking them in order to remove dirt and microscopic bacteria. Most people *don't* wash their raw cannabis prior to decarboxylation, but the more I read up on it, the more it makes sense to do so. Both hemp flower and marijuana buds contain sticky resin. Whether the plant was harvested in a large field or inside a grow facility, just about anything that was in the air, from pollen to dust, is probably stuck on that plant. Granted, most bacteria will likely be burnt off during the decarbing process. But if you have a pollen allergy, be aware that you might be baking pollen into your medication if you don't wash it first.

While some growers do have a washing process, it is not standard practice or required. I've found the best method from Jeff the 420 Chef, who recommends:

1. Prep: Break the hemp flower into popcorn-size pieces. Personally, I don't break the flower apart, as it can wind up in the final product if it gets too small during the infusion process. I do look for seeds and take them out (to plant later). I also remove any large stems. Most store-bought CBD hemp flower is already "prepped," so you can likely skip this step.

2. Soak: Place the hemp flower in a French press coffee maker and completely immerse in water. Distilled water is preferable. The hemp can be soaked for up to three days; change the water twice a day until it is clear. The reason to use a French press is that you can put the hemp flower at the bottom and press down on the plunger when you're ready to change the water. This keeps the flower from being thrown out with the dirty water, and it gently squeezes out the water each time.

3. Rinse: Transfer the hemp flower from the French press to a salad spinner. Spin for about 30 seconds to remove excess water. You don't need to worry about fully drying the hemp, as it will dry during the decarbing process.

4. Dry and Decarb: Preheat the oven to 240°F. Spread the hemp evenly on a rimmed baking sheet and cover loosely with aluminum foil; you can crimp the foil to the pan edges to hold in the odor. Bake for 1 to 1½ hours, until the hemp is completely dry. During this time, the hemp flower will go through the process of decarboxylation to "activate" the CBD in the raw plant (convert CBD-A to CBD).

QUICK HEMP FLOWER DECARBING. If you don't want to wait days to completely wash and decarb your hemp flower, Jeff the 420 Chef recommends a slightly faster process:

1. Soak the hemp flower overnight in distilled water.

2. The next day, drain the hemp in a fine-mesh strainer over the sink, then rinse with more distilled water.

3. Place the rinsed hemp flower in a large tea strainer (or tea infuser basket) or wrap it in cheesecloth. Bring filtered water to a boil in a saucepan and place the tea strainer with the hemp flower in the boiling water for 5 minutes.

4. Immediately remove after 5 minutes and place the tea strainer in ice water for 1 minute. Remove the tea strainer from the ice water and gently squeeze out excess water from the hemp. Next, remove the hemp flower from the strainer and spread it evenly on an oven-safe ceramic baking dish.

5. Preheat the oven to 300°F. Cover the hemp flower with foil and bake for 20 minutes.

DECARBING WITHOUT CLEANING THE HEMP FLOWER. If you want to forgo the cleaning, rinsing, straining, and squeezing process and go straight to decarbing your hemp, I recommend baking the hemp flower at 220°F for about 40 minutes or at 230°F for up to 30 minutes. The hemp will brown a bit as it cooks, but be sure to watch it—you don't want a black and burnt flower. You're looking for the buds to turn slightly brown and slightly crisp.

INFUSING CBD INTO COOKING OIL

You've now cleaned and decarbed your hemp, and it's ready for infusion. After the hemp flower has cooled following the decarboxylation process, you can use a French press to create a double boiler on the stovetop. Here's what you'll need:

- Hemp flower (decarboxylated)

- Cooking oil of choice: olive oil, coconut oil, hemp seed oil, etc.

- French press (4-cup capacity or larger)
- Cooking pot large enough to hold the French press
- Candy or instant-read thermometer
- Jar for storing the infused oil

You determine how much hemp flower to use according to the percentage of CBD in the flower. Find a formula that works for you so that it's easy to calculate how much CBD is in each meal and each serving. Typical ratios of hemp flower to oil are 2:1 or 1:1 (grams: fluid ounces). If hemp flower contains 24% CBD (approximately 215 to 240 milligrams per gram), some suggested ratios are 8 grams of CBD flower to 4 or 8 ounces of oil. Whatever you decide, you should also consider how the oil will *taste*. The more raw plant material added to a cup of oil, the greater the likelihood that you'll taste it in your food.

1. Place the decarbed CBD flower and 1 cup of cooking oil in a French press coffee maker. Put the lid on, but don't use the plunger yet.

2. Fill the cooking pot a quarter to halfway full of water and bring to a boil. The water should come slightly above the level of the cooking oil in the French press.

3. Stand the French press upright in the boiling water, essentially creating a double boiler. Place the thermometer in the water. The ideal temperature for infusing CBD into olive oil is around 200°F, so once the water is boiling, dial back the heat and simmer for 2 hours.

4. Check the water level every 20 minutes or so, refilling as necessary to maintain a constant level. Using oven mitts, lift the French press out of the water occasionally to give the oil a good stir, then set it back in the water.

5. After the oil has been simmering for 2 hours, carefully remove the French press from the water, using oven mitts. Press the plunger all the way down to strain the oil and keep the hemp flower and stray particles out of the final product.

6. Slowly pour the infused oil into a sterile jar or container with an airtight lid. Use a glass container such as a mason jar, or simply reuse the original oil container.

7. If you notice any particles in the oil, you can use cheesecloth to strain the oil again before using it. Store in a dark cabinet or pantry where the temperature is fairly consistent.

INFUSING CBD INTO BUTTER

You can use the same CBD ratio for butter as for cooking oil—such as 1 cup (2 sticks) butter to 4 to 8 grams CBD hemp flower. Remember, the more raw plant material you use, the more the butter (and any food made with it) is likely to taste like cannabis.

Unsalted organic butter yields the best results. Otherwise you can wind up with butter that has extra water pocketed somewhere in your silicone mold or container. Buying higher quality butter means less water in your butter, and that means a higher yield with higher potency. It's best to use butter that's already softened, so leave it at room temperature for a few hours prior to infusing.

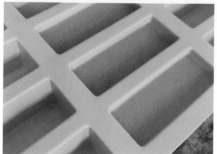

To make CBD butter, follow the same basic steps and use the same materials as for CBD cooking oil (above), but let the butter *simmer* for 3 hours. Don't let it boil, or it may burn.

Place 1 cup unsalted butter (2 sticks) in a French press. Every 20 minutes or so, lift it from the hot water to swirl the butter around. Be sure to watch the temperature on the candy thermometer— you'll want it to stay around 160°F, ideally, but never exceed 200°F.

Each rectangle of this silicone mold contains ¼ cup butter (4 tablespoons). To ensure that all the sticks are the same size, pour the butter into a measuring cup, then into the mold.

When finished with the infusion, refrigerate or freeze your CBD butter in an airtight container or silicone mold.

MAKING CBD BUTTER IN THE OVEN

Making CBD butter in the oven saves you from worrying about burning your butter or maintaining consistent heat on the stovetop. You can also make a larger batch this way. Here's what you need:

- hemp flower (decarboxylated)
- 2 cups (4 sticks) unsalted butter, softened
- square or rectangular oven-safe dish

- silicone spatula
- cheesecloth, fine-mesh sieve, or tea strainer
- jar or silicone mold for storing infused butter

1. Preheat the oven to 225°F.

2. Combine the hemp and butter in the oven-safe dish (2 cups butter and 4 to 8 grams of hemp flower, or whatever ratio works best for you). Place in the oven.

3. Once the butter has melted, stir with the spatula to make sure the hemp is completely submerged in the butter. Bake for 4 hours, stirring once an hour.

4. Remove from the oven and strain the butter to remove the flower particles, using cheesecloth, a sieve, or a tea strainer. Or you can pour it into a French press to strain it—the mesh on the plunger should be fine enough to capture the particles.

5. Once all the particles are deposited in the cheesecloth/sieve, press down with the spatula or with your hand to squeeze out all the butter you can.

6. Store in an airtight container or silicone mold in the refrigerator or freezer.

CANNABIS INFUSION MACHINES

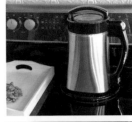

If you're worried about your hemp flower losing its potency as it is infused into butter or oil, you can purchase a Magical Butter or LEVO infusion machine to take out the guesswork. Here are the benefits of going with a machine to create your CBD butter or oil:

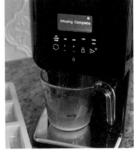

- The machine does the work for you. You literally put the hemp flower and oil/butter into the machine and just wait for it to be done.

- The machine heats the CBD at the right temperatures and makes sure the medication is consistent throughout the entire batch.

- There's less cleanup required.

- The house won't smell like pot at all. If you've made cannabutter, you know the smell is quite strong and will soon move beyond the kitchen, even if you have the stove exhaust fan going at full blast.

- The infused butter and oil have a better taste, in my opinion—more refined and less earthy.

Magical Butter Machine (top) and the LEVO II (bottom)

- These machines can easily infuse food and drink products with cannabis, so you can make a variety of recipes without using extra pots or pans.

- The machines are inconspicuous. The Magical Butter Machine looks like a large stainless-steel electric kettle for boiling water. The LEVO looks like a Keurig or espresso machine.

The **Magical Butter Machine (MBM)** can infuse up to 5 cups of oil or butter at a time, so you can make a big batch of butter and freeze it for use later. It also has a non-heat option, so you can use it as a blender. You do have to strain the infused butter or oil through cheesecloth, so there is still some mess involved, but you don't have to stand over a hot pan to constantly move the butter or oil to make sure it's infusing properly.

The **LEVO II** is my new favorite kitchen gadget because it has a function to *decarb* the hemp flower before infusing it. The LEVO can make up to 2 cups of oil or butter at a time. That's less than the MBM, but 2 cups are more than enough for a day's cooking. The LEVO is designed for cooking with hemp flower and other herbs so it doesn't exceed 200°F. I like to experiment by adding flavors such as garlic and rosemary to small batches; if the flavors come out too light or too strong, I can make another batch and marry the two. And what I really like is how easy it is to clean—everything goes in the dishwasher. Also, there's no straining through cheesecloth; the machine dispenses clear oil and butter with the touch of a button. There's also an app with recipes and time/temp indicators that you can access from your phone.

HERB INFUSIONS WITH CBD BUTTER/CBD OIL

Some of the recipes in this book call for CBD butter or oil infused with herbs. Here are a couple of combinations that you can use as is or vary with your own choice of herbs. Simply add the herbs in with the hemp flower as you infuse so that the herbs and the hemp can be strained together.

CBD CHIVE BUTTER WITH GARLIC AND THYME

- 1 cup (2 sticks) unsalted butter
- 4 to 7 grams hemp flower
- 3 tablespoons loosely packed chopped fresh chives
- 1 clove garlic, minced
- 1 tablespoon loosely packed chopped thyme

CBD ROSEMARY COOKING OIL

- 1 cup oil of choice
- 4 to 7 grams hemp flower
- ¼ cup loosely packed fresh rosemary leaves, without stems

The benefit of using vegetable or refined coconut oil as a base is that it doesn't have a distinct taste, so it can be used in just about any recipe. However, coconut oil does congeal at cold temperatures, so it can change the consistency of a meal if you refrigerate leftovers. If you like the nutritional benefits of hemp seed oil (which can be used in foods meant to be kept chilled, such as mayonnaise) but don't like its taste, infusing rosemary or other herbs in addition to the CBD will help.

CBD-INFUSED CONDIMENTS

To add CBD to condiments such as honey, maple syrup, or ketchup, it's best to heat the condiment first. Since cannabinoids bind best with fat, I find that the best way to put CBD into a condiment that doesn't contain a fat- or an oil-based ingredient is with water-soluble CBD. That way the CBD will be mixed evenly throughout the condiment.

You can also opt to add water-soluble CBD to an individual serving of practically any kind of food. This means that you can cook a meal *without* CBD and then add a dose to your own portion.

DON'T OVERCOOK IT!

If you've ever cooked with marijuana, you know that THC burns off at a different temperature than CBD does. THC is completely degraded at temperatures above 392°F and starts to break down long before that. Similarly, CBD will begin to evaporate as it heats, which means less potency in your food. Whether you're adding a small amount or opting for a stronger dose, all the CBD will degrade at the same rate and in the same temperature range.

The boiling point of CBD is between 320°F and 356°F. It's best not to heat CBD for too long at 350°F. To be safe, stick with a temperature no higher than 340°F. Frying or sautéing with CBD butter or CBD oil also increases the likelihood that the CBD will lose its potency, since the CBD is directly in contact with the pan's hot surface. High heat can also bring out CBD's bitterness.

When I bake with CBD, I like to keep the temperature at or below 325°F and use recipes that call for a cooking time of one hour or less. However, you *can* bake cookies, brownies, and breads at 350°F, since the internal temperature of baked goods will be lower than the external temperature of the oven.

MAKING CBD-INFUSED BUTTER WITHOUT HEMP FLOWER

You can infuse butter—or cooking oil, or any food or drink item—with CBD oil or CBD powder, readily purchased in a store or online. Here's what you'll need:

- 2 cups (4 sticks) unsalted butter, cut into smaller pieces
- 4 cups water
- 10 grams pure CBD oil

1. Combine the butter pieces, water, and CBD oil in a medium saucepan.

2. Cook uncovered over low heat for 3 to 4 hours.

3. Using a metal spoon, gently stir every 30 minutes. The mixture will thicken as the water cooks off. Don't allow it to boil as this could decrease the amount of CBD.

4. Once the mixture is glossy and dense, remove it from the stovetop and let cool.

5. When the mixture has cooled, pour it into an airtight container. Secure the lid firmly and place the container in the refrigerator for at least 2 hours to let the butter solidify. Store it in the refrigerator until you're ready to use.

MAKING CBD-INFUSED COOKING OIL WITHOUT HEMP FLOWER

CBD crystals or the powdered form of CBD can be infused into cooking oil. Manufacturers often recommended starting with an initial dose of 5 to 10 milligrams. Here's what you'll need:

- 1 cup cooking oil (coconut, olive, canola, etc.)
- 1 gram crushed CBD crystals or CBD powder

1. Pour the oil into a medium saucepan and heat on the stovetop at the lowest temperature; bring to a simmer but do not allow to boil.

2. Add the CBD crystals or powder and stir until completely dissolved.

3. Place a candy thermometer in the oil; the temperature shouldn't exceed 245°F or the CBD will burn and you'll be left with just oil.

4. Once the CBD is dissolved, remove from the heat and let cool, then pour the CBD-infused oil into a glass jar and secure the lid. Store at room temperature.

***

For each recipe in this book, there's a suggested amount of CBD to incorporate and instructions for when to incorporate it in the cooking process. Whenever possible, I give multiple options for the source of CBD (water-soluble CBD, CBD butter, CBD coconut oil, etc.) so you can choose what works best for you. I recommend that you determine your daily dose of CBD before cooking with it, if possible. That way you won't waste any CBD by cooking with way too much or cooking with way too little (so that it has no effect).

The recipes in this book typically contain .5 to 1 milliliter of water-soluble CBD per serving. While everyone's ailments are different and a daily amount of CBD varies from person to person, it's not uncommon for people to take 1 to 2 milliliters of water-soluble CBD per day, so incorporating CBD into two meals or drinks per day could be sufficient. Most of the recipes are for one or two servings, and easy to double or triple to make family-size amounts. The smaller serving sizes can also come in handy if the CBD does wind up overpowering the flavor of the meal. It's definitely possible to add too much CBD to a recipe, so instead of wasting your medication (and your time and the meal you just prepared), you can simply double the recipe to dilute the taste and freeze or refrigerate leftovers for later. You can also opt to make these recipes without CBD and then add doses to individual portions, making the food easily shareable. And many of the meals include sauces, so you can top off one of your own recipes with a CBD sauce from this book. Remember that simply adding a store-bought water-soluble CBD or CBD oil to your meal is often the easiest solution.

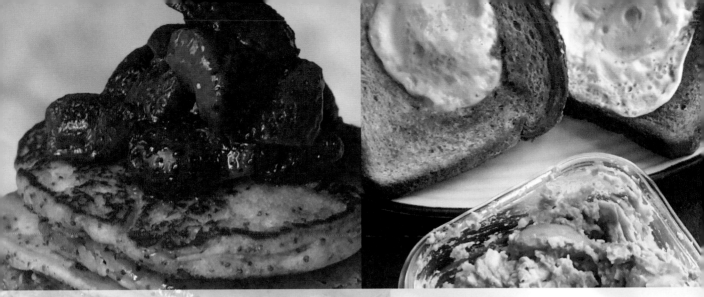

Chapter **2**

BREAKFAST & BRUNCH

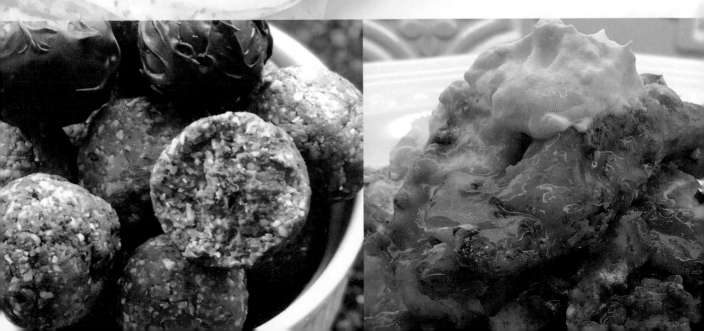

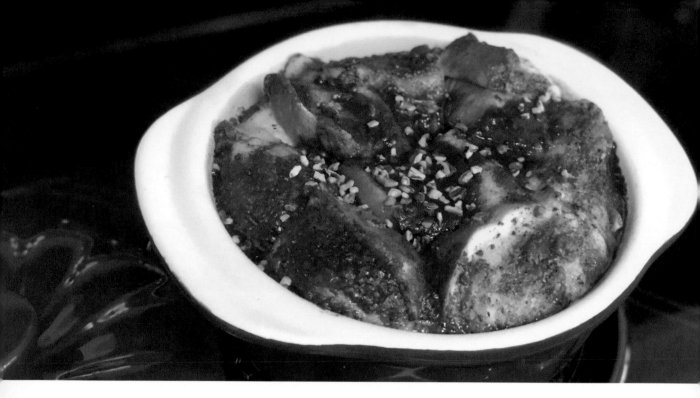

MAKE-AHEAD
FRENCH TOAST SOUFFLÉ

This is a great recipe for busy mornings. It's also my favorite way to use a loaf of bread that's a little stale or would otherwise go to waste. Everything can be assembled the night before, or the topping can be made in the morning while the soufflé is in the oven. This is the fluffiest of French toasts and a delicious, easy breakfast that also makes an impressive dessert. The recipe calls for half of a loaf of sandwich bread; most sandwich bread comes in a package of 22 slices, but you can use any type of bread (wheat, white, etc). I've also used half a loaf of French bread cut thin, or you can double the recipe for a full loaf.

Prep time: 10 minutes | **Chill time:** at least 4 hours | **Bake time:** 45 minutes | **Makes:** 2 to 4 servings

SOUFFLÉ

½ loaf of sandwich bread (10 to 12 pieces)

½ cup chopped pecans

4 large eggs

1 cup whole milk or half-and-half

1 teaspoon vanilla extract

½ teaspoon salt

1 teaspoon ground cinnamon

¼ teaspoon ground nutmeg

CINNAMON TOPPING

4 tablespoons unsalted butter, melted

½ cup brown sugar

1 teaspoon ground cinnamon

½ teaspoon ground nutmeg

ACCOMPANIMENT

Dulce de Leche as syrup (page 110)

CHOOSE ONE OF THE FOLLOWING CBD OPTIONS:
For the 4 tablespoons of butter in the topping, substitute one of the following:

- 1 milliliter water-soluble CBD mixed into 4 tablespoons melted butter (recommended)
- 1 tablespoon CBD butter + 3 tablespoons unmedicated butter
- 2 tablespoons CBD butter + 2 tablespoons unmedicated butter

---

1. For the fluffiest soufflé, use a small soufflé or casserole dish (about 1½-quart). Cut the bread slices into quarters and arrange in the baking dish in overlapping layers along with the pecans. In a medium bowl, whisk together the eggs, milk, vanilla, salt, cinnamon, and nutmeg.*

2. Pour the egg mixture over the bread, then cover and refrigerate for 4 to 6 hours or overnight to allow the bread to soak up the egg mixture.

3. When ready to bake, preheat the oven to 350°F.

4. While the oven heats, prepare the cinnamon topping. Melt the butter in the microwave or on the stovetop and then mix in the brown sugar, cinnamon, and nutmeg.

5. Spread 1 to 2 tablespoons of the topping over the soufflé, then cover the dish with a lid or foil. Bake for 25 to 30 minutes, then uncover and bake for 15 minutes more, until the top layer is fluffy.

6. Meanwhile, heat ½ to 1 cup of the Dulce de Leche and mix in the remaining cinnamon topping, using an emulsion blender if you have one.

7. Remove the soufflé from the oven and cut in slices. Serve with the Dulce de Leche syrup.

I like to make the CBD-infused topping first and then "butter" the bread slices with it before cutting and layering them in the baking dish. This enhances the flavor of the soufflé and distributes the CBD throughout. There'll still be enough topping left to add to the top after the soufflé chills.

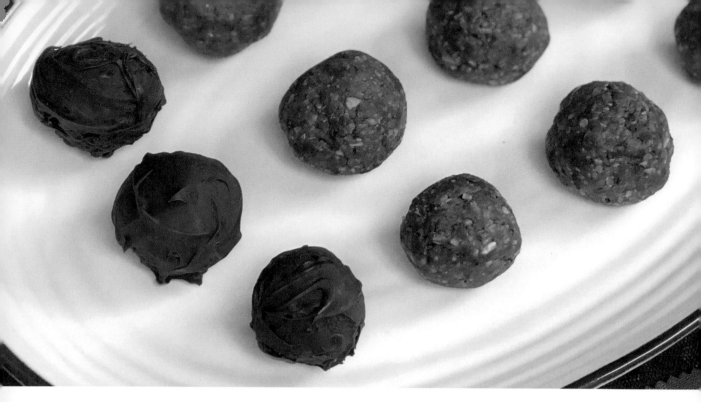

NO-BAKE CARAMEL PUMPKIN SPICE ENERGY BITES

If you're the type of person who skips breakfast or isn't very hungry in the morning, grab a few of these little energy bites as you're headed out the door to get the day started. When it comes to nutrition, they are packed! Rolled oats contain soluble fiber, which helps you feel full longer. And hemp and pumpkin are superfoods. Pumpkin is full of iron, zinc, vitamin C, several B vitamins, beta carotene (what our bodies process into vitamin A), potassium, and fiber. Hemp has many of the same nutritional benefits and is also a complete source of protein (all nine essential amino acids), plus fiber, vitamin E, magnesium, phosphorous, and potassium.

If you want to make a simpler version, just leave out the maca powder, MCT oil, and syrup/honey. Maca powder—made from the maca root, native to Peru—can improve energy and stamina without the jitters and crashes of caffeine, but it has a malty taste that can overpower other flavors. You can also add more maca, but taste first. I recommend adding ½ teaspoon at a time, going up to as much as 1 tablespoon. Most grocery stores sell maca powder in the health food or vitamin and supplement aisle; it's usually found near the protein powder, MCT oil, and hemp seeds, but it can also be purchased online from a variety of sites (even Amazon).

I like to store my Caramel Pumpkin Spice Energy Bites in silicone ice cube trays so that they take up very little room in my refrigerator or freezer. The CBD coconut oil helps keep the balls compact.

These pair well with yogurt, too. And for extra sweetness and crunch, you can coat the bites in melted chocolate after they've been chilled.

Prep time: 15 minutes | **Chill time:** about 1 hour | **Makes:** about 30 bites

2 cups rolled oats

½ cup canned pumpkin purée

1 teaspoon MCT oil

½ cup CBD Dulce de Leche (page 110)

¼ cup maple syrup or honey

½ teaspoon pumpkin pie spice or ground cinnamon

¼ cup hemp seeds or hemp protein powder

1 teaspoon maca powder

½ teaspoon vanilla extract

½ cup dark chocolate chips

CBD OPTION
• **1 to 2 tablespoons CBD coconut oil**

1. Place the rolled oats in a blender or food processor and pulse to a flour-like consistency.

2. Place 1 cup of the oat flour in a large bowl; add the pumpkin purée, MCT oil, CBD Dulce de Leche, maple syrup or honey, pumpkin pie spice, hemp seeds or hemp protein powder, maca powder, vanilla, and CBD coconut oil, if using. Stir with a spoon or spatula; use your hands to mix further until well combined.

3. Add the remaining oat flour, ¼ cup at a time. The mixture should be moist and slightly sticky.

4. Place the chocolate chips in a blender or food processor and pulse into small pieces. Add to the pumpkin mixture, combining well.

5. Scoop the mixture out with your hands or a spoon and use your hands to roll into balls slightly smaller than a golf ball (think party-size meatball appetizer).

6. Freeze 1 hour or until solid, then store in the freezer or refrigerator for up to a week.

BENEFITS OF MCT OIL

Medium-chain triglyceride (MCT) oil is yet another ingredient known to provide energy. It can also help with weight loss, appetite control, and inflammation. Usually made from coconut or palm kernel oil, MCT oil is flavorless, so it can be added to just about anything. This can be found in any grocery store in the health food/supplement section.

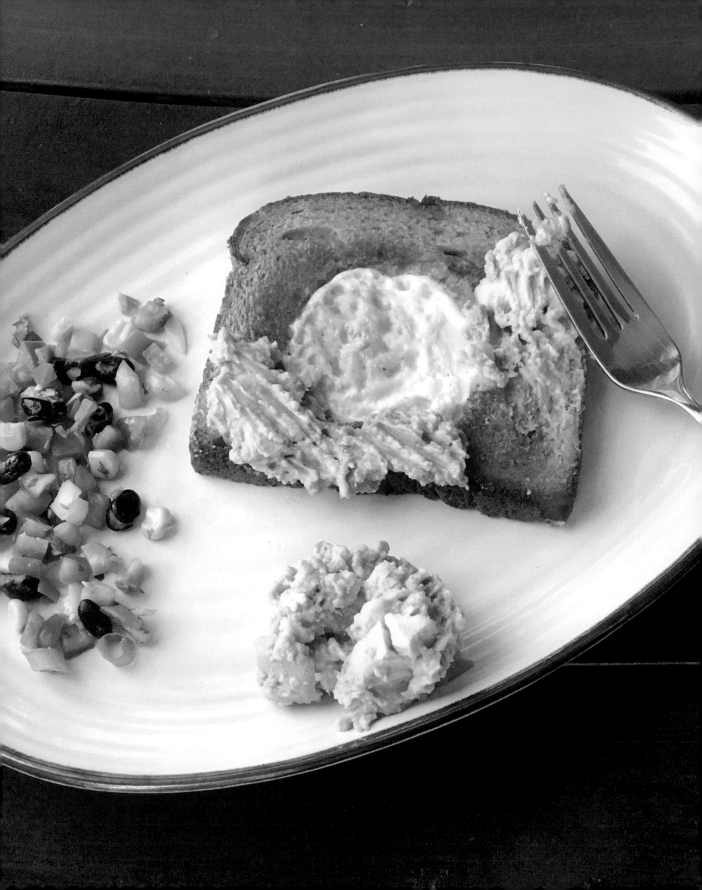

EGG-IN-THE-BASKET AVOCADO TOAST

When I lived in Northern California, we had quite a number of hens to provide us with eggs every day for breakfast. Egg-in-the-basket toast was my go-to solution for a quick and healthy breakfast, and adding the avocado is a fun twist. Avocados contain 20 different vitamins and minerals, including vitamin E and more vitamin K and potassium than bananas—great brain food to start the day! You can switch up the garnishes on the toast to keep the flavors unique each day.

Prep and cook time: 15 minutes | **Makes:** 1 serving

1 slice bread

1 ripe avocado, halved and pitted

1 tablespoon butter, or more as needed

1 egg

CBD butter, if needed (optional)

salt, pepper, and favorite garnishes (such as cilantro, parsley, shredded cheese, pico de gallo)

CHOOSE ONE OF THE FOLLOWING CBD OPTIONS:
- **.5 to 1 milliliter water-soluble CBD (recommended)**
- **1½ teaspoons CBD olive oil**

1. Toast the bread in a toaster.

2. Use a spoon to scoop the avocado meat into a bowl.

3. Add the CBD option of choice and mash with a fork until well blended, then set aside while you cook the egg.

4. Cut a hole in the center of the toasted bread, large enough to contain the egg. (A small cookie cutter or the rim of a drinking glass works well for making the hole.)

5. Melt the butter in a nonstick skillet or griddle over medium-high heat. Rub both sides of the toast on the melted butter, then place the toast in the center of the skillet.

6. Crack the egg and slowly pour it into the hole in the bread. It will start to cook immediately. Adding the egg slowly keeps it within the hole as it cooks and lets it fry to a slight crispiness.

7. Cook to your preferred level of doneness, 1 to 2 minutes. If you wish, add more butter to the skillet and flip the toast over to finish cooking the egg.

8. Transfer to a plate and butter the toast with CBD butter, if you wish.

9. Top with the mashed CBD avocado and additional garnishes, as desired.

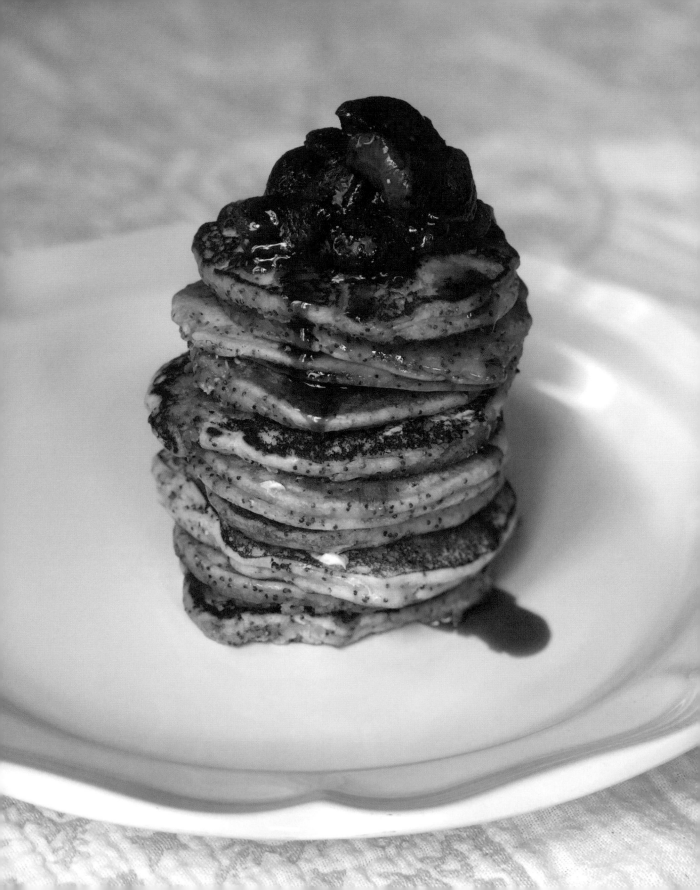

LEMON POPPY SEED PANCAKES

These pancakes are perfect for a weekend brunch. For variety, you can experiment with the flavor of the yogurt that goes into the batter. Honey and vanilla complement the other ingredients, but lemon or strawberry yogurt could be a nice touch as well.

This vegan batter is a bit stickier than traditional pancake batter—to keep it from sticking to the griddle, you may want to wet your pancake turner under cold water before flipping the pancake.

Prep and cook time: 20 minutes | **Makes:** about 15 to 20 pancakes

1½ cups self-rising flour (or add ½ teaspoon baking soda to regular flour)

1 tablespoon poppy seeds

½ cup dairy-free milk (sweetened vanilla almond milk or hemp milk)

1 teaspoon vanilla extract

¼ cup (4 tablespoons) flavored yogurt (I prefer honey vanilla yogurt)

5 tablespoons maple syrup

juice and zest of 1 medium lemon (about 3 tablespoons juice and 1 teaspoon zest)

½ teaspoon lemon extract

accompaniments of choice—Strawberry Syrup (page 113), CBD butter, Homemade Whipped Cream (page 72), or Dulce de Leche (page 110)

CHOOSE ONE OF THE FOLLOWING CBD OPTIONS
- **1 to 2 tablespoons CBD vegetable oil or coconut oil**
- **2 milliliters water-soluble CBD**

1. Grease a griddle or nonstick pan with cooking spray or a little vegetable oil. Heat on low heat for about 10 minutes (approximately the amount of time it takes to mix the ingredients).

2. Mix the flour, baking soda (if using), and poppy seeds in a large bowl.

3. In another bowl, mix together the milk, vanilla, yogurt, maple syrup, lemon juice and zest, lemon extract, and CBD. Combine well; the mixture will be runny but thick.

4. Slowly add the wet ingredients to the dry ingredients, mixing until well combined.

5. For each pancake, add ¼ cup batter to the heated pan or griddle and cook for about 30 seconds, then flip to the other side and cook for 30 seconds more.

6. Remove from pan and serve with Strawberry Syrup or other toppings of choice.

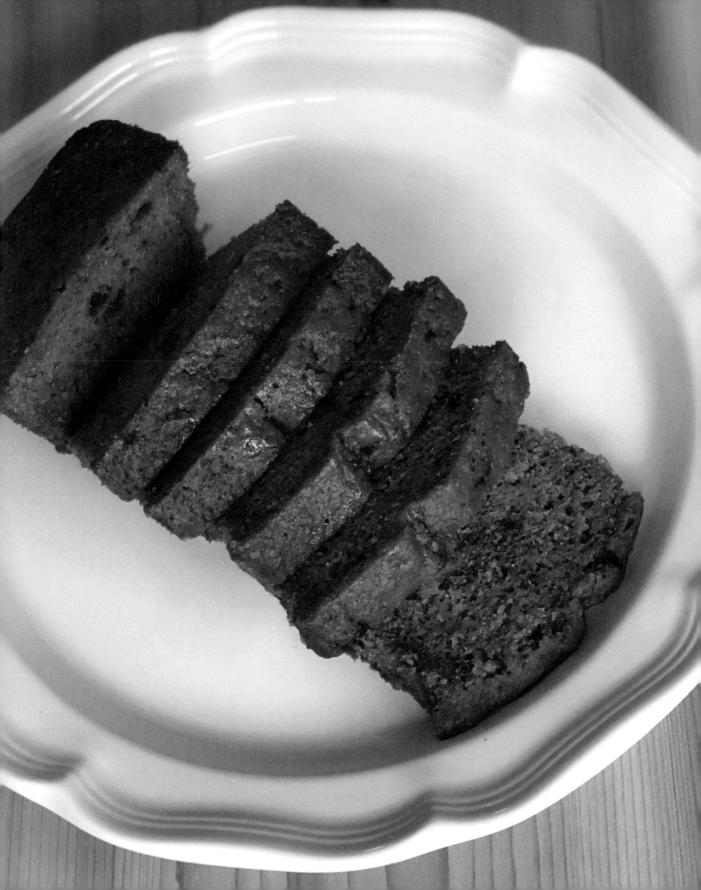

STRAWBERRY BREAD

This one of my favorite recipes passed down to me by my mother (thanks, Mom!). The bread is moist and delightful on its own or with a smear of cream cheese. This recipe is easily modified to make strawberry muffins; just prep a muffin tin with muffin liners and pour in the batter, leaving some space for the muffins to rise. Bake for up to 1 hour.

Prep and cook time: 1 hour 20 minutes | **Makes:** 1 loaf (8 to 10 pieces)

1 (10-ounce) package frozen strawberries packed in syrup, thawed but not drained

2 eggs

¾ cup vegetable oil

1½ cups all-purpose flour

1 cup sugar

1 teaspoon ground cinnamon

½ teaspoon baking soda

CHOOSE ONE OF THE FOLLOWING CBD OPTIONS
Instead of the ¾ cup of vegetable oil, use one of the following:

- ¼ cup CBD cooking oil (preferably vegetable oil) + ½ cup unmedicated vegetable oil

- ½ cup CBD cooking oil + ¼ cup unmedicated vegetable oil

- ½ cup vegetable oil + ¼ cup combined CBD and unmedicated vegetable oil (1 to 3 tablespoons CBD cooking oil, the remainder unmedicated vegetable oil)

Or, instead of the above, add 5 milliliters of water-soluble CBD before blending in Step 2.

1. Preheat the oven to 325°F. Grease a 9x5-inch loaf pan; place parchment paper on the bottom to ensure the bread won't stick to the pan.

2. Purée the strawberries in a blender. Add the eggs, oil, and CBD and blend well.

3. Sift the flour, sugar, cinnamon, and baking soda into a large bowl. Make a well in the center of the dry ingredients and pour in the strawberry purée mixture.

4. Mix until well combined, then pour into the prepared pan.

5. Bake for 1 hour 10 minutes; or stick a toothpick into the center of the bread to check that it is no longer wet.

6. Let cool completely on a rack before removing from the pan. Flip the bread out of the pan by inverting it. You can run a knife around the edges of the bread to loosen it from the sides to help pop it out.

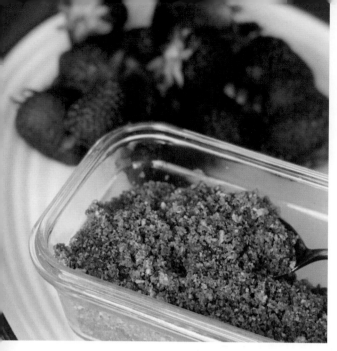

GRAHAM CRACKER CRUMBLE

Pair this Graham Cracker Crumble with Dulce de Leche (page 110) to make a sensational topping for yogurt or desserts. It's also great as a crust for the Peanut Butter Mousse (page 69) or the Chocolate Mousse (page 71).

Total time: 10 min |
Makes: 6 to 10 servings

1 tablespoon hemp seeds

¼ cup sugar

1 tablespoon unsweetened cocoa powder

¼ cup (4 tablespoons) unsalted butter, or more if needed

1¼ cups crushed graham crackers

¾ cup crushed ginger snaps

CHOOSE ONE OF THESE CBD OPTIONS
Instead of the ¼ cup of unsalted butter, use one of the following:

• 2 tablespoons CBD-infused coconut oil + 2 tablespoons unmedicated butter

• 2 tablespoons CBD butter + 2 tablespoons unmedicated butter

1. In a blender or food processor, crush the graham crackers, ginger snaps, and hemp seeds until fully combined and granulated, then mix in the sugar and cocoa powder.

2. Transfer the mixture to a medium bowl.

3. Melt the butter in a medium saucepan and add to the graham cracker mixture along with the CBD. Use your fingers to bind the butter to the graham cracker crumbles. The mixture should be slightly moist; you can choose to add additional butter if necessary. Transfer to a covered container and refrigerate.

4. Use as a topping for a yogurt parfait or as an ingredient in No-Bake Caramel Pumpkin Spice Energy Bites (page 22).

COOKING *with* **CBD**

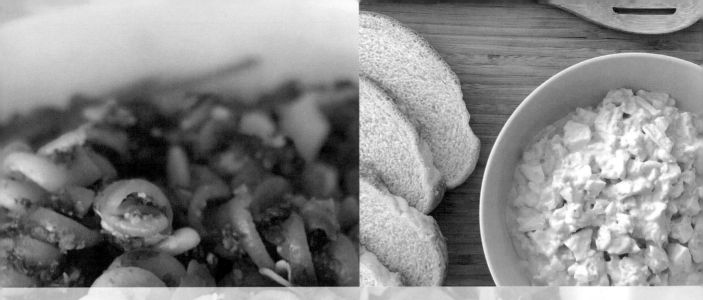

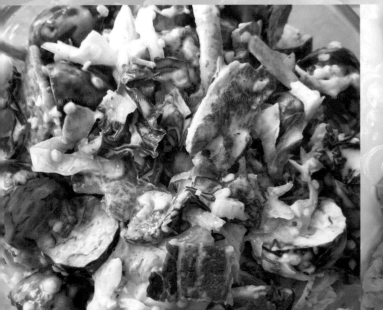

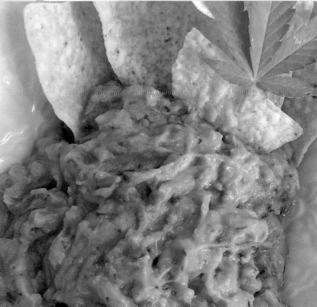

Chapter **3**

LUNCH

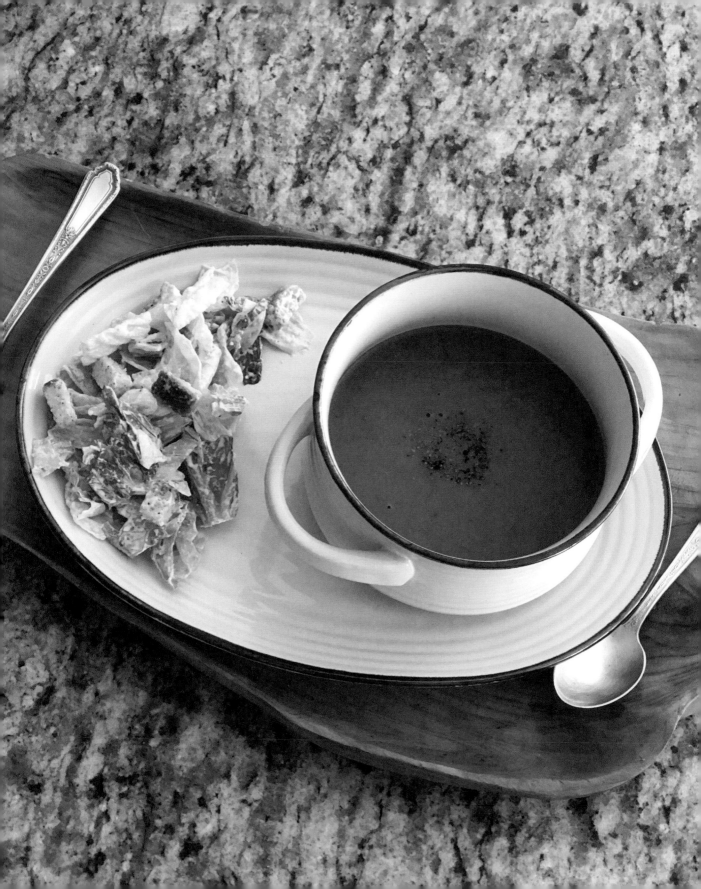

HEARTY FIRE-ROASTED TOMATO SOUP

This is a phenomenally creamy vegan tomato soup. Although I love my immersion blender, when blending soups I prefer to use a large blender with a lid. I find that this mixes in the CBD better—and I make much less of a mess when I can put a lid on what I'm blending.

Total time: 20 minutes | **Makes:** 6 to 8 servings

1 tablespoon olive oil

1 small white onion, diced

4 cloves garlic, minced

2 stems fresh thyme

2 (14-ounce) cans fire-roasted diced tomatoes, or diced tomatoes of choice

2 cups chicken or vegetable stock

2 teaspoons Italian seasoning

1 tablespoon honey or brown sugar

⅓ cup chopped fresh basil leaves (or 1 tablespoon dried basil leaves)

salt and pepper (freshly ground pepper if possible)

freshly grated Parmesan cheese or chopped fresh basil, for topping

CHOOSE ONE OF THE FOLLOWING CBD OPTIONS
- 2 tablespoons CBD cooking oil (rosemary olive oil preferred)
- 2 to 4 milliliters water-soluble CBD

1. Heat the olive oil in a large saucepan over medium high heat. Add the onion and sauté on medium high for 4 to 5 minutes, stirring, until soft and translucent.

2. Add the garlic and thyme and sauté for 1 to 2 minutes, stirring, until fragrant.

3. Stir in the tomatoes, stock, Italian seasoning, honey or brown sugar, and basil.

4. When the soup reaches a simmer, reduce the heat to medium low.

5. Cover with a lid that is slightly ajar and simmer for another 5 to 10 minutes.

6. Uncover and purée the soup until smooth, using an immersion or regular blender or a food processor. Add the CBD as you blend.

7. Season with salt and pepper to taste. Serve immediately, topped with grated Parmesan or chopped basil.

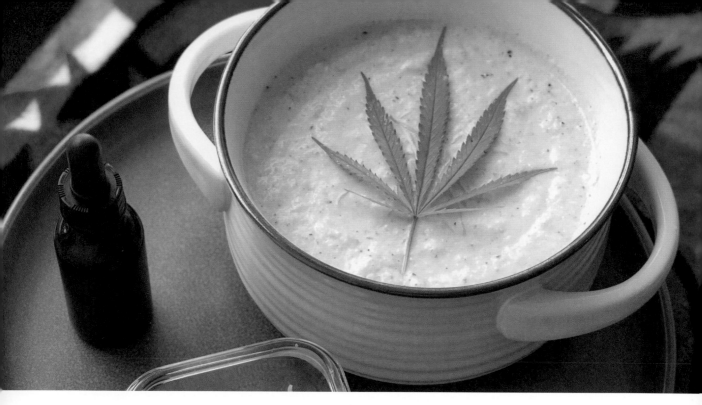

CREAMY CAULIFLOWER HEMP SOUP

I like to include cheddar cheese and bacon in this soup, but these can easily be left out to make it vegan. To save time, I use frozen riced cauliflower; there's a medley with carrots and extra vegetables that tastes great in the soup. You can also add cooked corn to make this into a creamy corn chowder. If you have leftovers, the soup can be frozen to be reheated another day.

Prep and cook time: 30 minutes | Makes: up to 4 bowls

2 tablespoons olive oil

1 teaspoon minced garlic or ½ teaspoon garlic powder

2 stems fresh thyme

5 strips cooked bacon, chopped, plus extra for serving (optional)

1 cauliflower head, chopped or riced (1½ cups), or 1 (16-ounce) bag frozen riced cauliflower

1½ cups vegetable broth

¼ cup hemp seeds

¼ cup lemon juice, from 2 medium lemons

1 teaspoon salt

¼ teaspoon pepper

¼ teaspoon garlic powder

½ teaspoon onion powder

½ cup freshly grated Parmesan or vegan cheese (optional)

2 tablespoons softened CBD Chive Butter with Garlic and Thyme (page 16)

cheddar cheese, for serving (optional)

COOKING *with* CBD

1. In a large pot, warm the olive oil over medium-low heat; add the minced garlic or ½ teaspoon garlic powder, thyme, and bacon (if using). Cook 1 to 2 minutes, stirring, until the ingredients are fragrant.

2. Add the cauliflower, stirring to combine.

3. Pour in the vegetable broth and bring to a boil.

4. Reduce to a simmer, cover with a lid, and cook for up to 10 minutes.

5. If using raw chopped cauliflower, make sure it is tender enough to mash with a spoon. Then remove the mixture from the heat and set aside.

6. In a blender, combine the hemp seeds, lemon juice, salt and pepper, garlic powder, and onion powder.

7. Transfer the cauliflower broth to the blender. Add Parmesan or vegan cheese (if using) and CBD; blend until smooth and creamy.

8. Serve immediately or return to the stove to heat slightly and melt the Parmesan further before serving.

9. Add additional bacon, cheddar cheese, or other garnishes to taste.

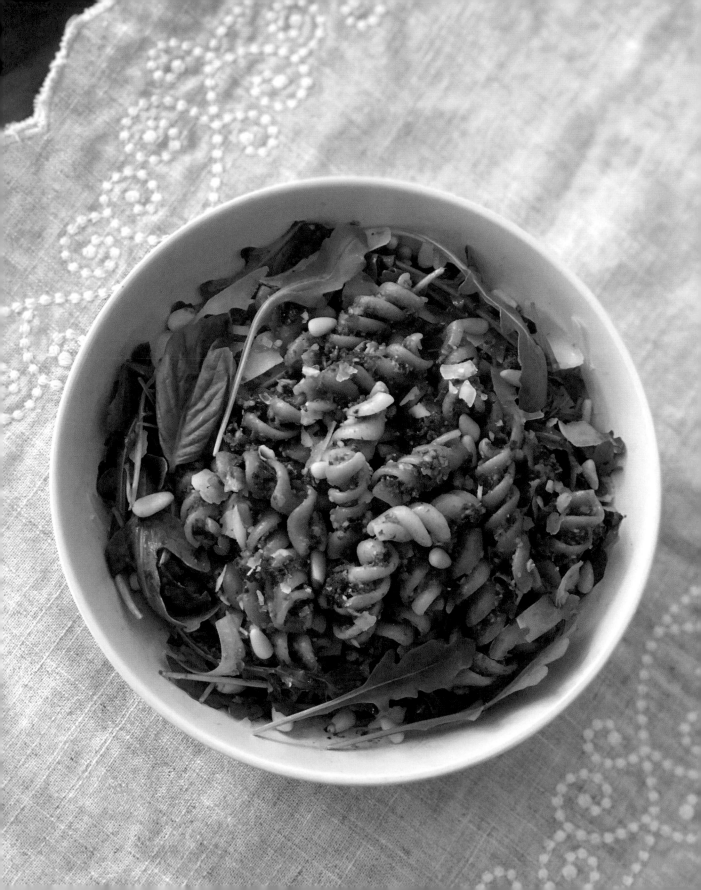

SUN-DRIED TOMATO PESTO PASTA WITH ARUGULA

Easy 20-minute healthy lunch! This can be made in advance and refrigerated overnight; it can be served cold or at room temperature. Personally, I prefer it warm and freshly made. The heat really activates the flavors of all the ingredients.

Depending on the shape and size of your pasta, you might not need a full 8-ounce package. I used 3 cups of vegetable pasta to make 3 servings for this dish.

Prep and cook time: 20 minutes | **Makes:** 2 to 3 servings

salt

8 ounces dried pasta (gluten-free, vegetable, egg noodle, or whatever you choose, but pasta with grooves works best)

3 ounces (1 cup) sun-dried tomatoes (not in oil)

2 tablespoons CBD olive oil

1 cup chopped fresh basil, plus more for topping

4 cloves garlic, minced

2 tablespoons grated Parmesan cheese, plus more for topping

1 cup loosely packed arugula

3 tablespoons hemp seeds, plus more for topping

3 tablespoons toasted pine nuts (optional)

CBD OPTION
- Instead of the 2 tablespoons of CBD olive oil, use unmedicated olive oil and add 2 to 3 milliliters of water-soluble CBD.

1. In a large saucepan, bring water to a boil, add salt and pasta, and cook according to package instructions.

2. Meanwhile, in a food processor or blender, combine the sun-dried tomatoes, CBD olive oil, basil, garlic, and 2 tablespoons of Parmesan cheese and blend to a pesto-like consistency. If the mixture seems too dry, add a little hot pasta water (2 to 3 tablespoons). It doesn't have to have a finely pureed consistency, just enough to blend the ingredients.

3. Drain the cooked pasta in a colander and return it to the hot saucepan.

4. Add the sun-dried tomato pesto and toss until the pasta is fully coated, then add the arugula.

5. Garnish as desired with hemp seeds, grated Parmesan, chopped basil, and pine nuts. Serve warm.

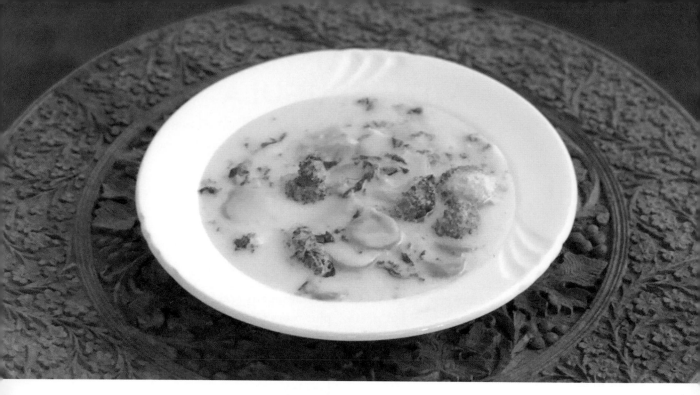

HOMESTYLE BROCCOLI CHEDDAR SOUP

The flavor of the cheese is really important for the taste of the soup. Pick a sharp cheddar that you really enjoy. You can use store-bought cheese that's already grated, but it will be milder and less cheesy. You can also use frozen veggies to save time. I'm not the biggest fan of broccoli, so I don't add the stems, and I've also made the soup with only 1 cup of bite-size pieces of broccoli florets and that's still enough for me, especially with the kale included. I also like to slice the carrots very fine on my vegetable mandoline (about 1/16-inch thick). You can use regular CBD butter instead of the chive version, but the fragrant smell that comes from the carrots, thyme, and CBD Chive Butter with Garlic and Thyme is seriously mouthwatering.

Total time: 30 minutes | **Makes:** 6 to 8 servings

¼ cup CBD Chive Butter with Garlic and Thyme (page 16)

2 medium carrots, diced

2 stems fresh thyme (optional)

5 strips cooked bacon, chopped fine, plus extra for serving (optional)

1 teaspoon garlic powder

1 tablespoon onion powder

3 cups vegetable stock or chicken stock (or bouillon cubes)

¼ cup all-purpose flour

2 cups milk or half-and-half

½ teaspoon paprika (optional)

1 teaspoon Dijon mustard or ½ teaspoon dry mustard powder

1 large head broccoli, florets chopped small (about 2 to 3 cups, or up to 4 cups if chopped stems are included)

8 ounces (2 cups) freshly grated sharp cheddar cheese, plus extra for serving

1 cup finely chopped kale (optional)

1 teaspoon salt, or as needed

½ teaspoon freshly ground pepper, or as needed

CBD OPTIONS
Instead of ¼ cup of CBD Chive Butter with Garlic and Thyme, use one of the following:

- 2 tablespoons CBD Chive Butter with Garlic and Thyme + 2 tablespoons unmedicated butter

- 2 tablespoons unmedicated butter + 2 tablespoons CBD cooking oil (olive or coconut)

- ¼ cup unmedicated butter + 4 to 6 milliliters water-soluble CBD (add in Step 7)

1. In a large pot over medium heat, stir together the CBD Chive Butter with Garlic and Thyme, carrots, thyme, and bacon until the butter is softened or gently melted and fragrant.

2. Stir in the garlic powder and onion powder.

3. Stir in the stock, flour, milk, paprika, and mustard and whisk until well combined.

4. Continue cooking the soup, stirring occasionally, until it reaches a simmer. Reduce heat to low.

5. Add the broccoli, cheese, and kale. Continue cooking for 2 to 4 minutes, until the broccoli is tender. Stir frequently to keep a "skin" from forming on the top.

6. Add the salt and pepper; taste and add more if needed.

7. Allow to cool slightly before serving so that the soup thickens a bit more. Water-soluble CBD can be added at this time (be sure to mix well). Can also add shredded cheese and bacon as garnishes.

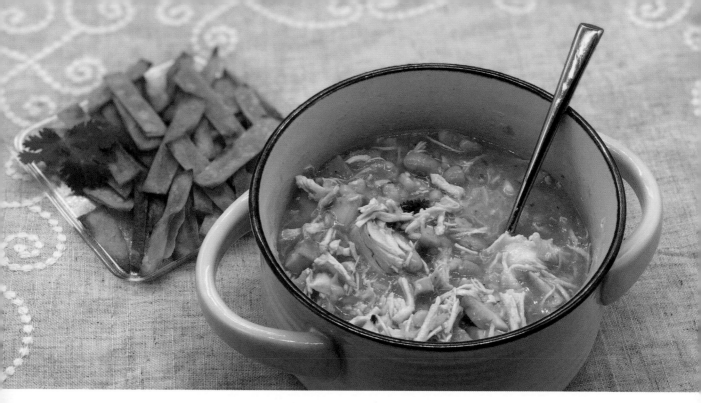

CHICKEN CHILI TORTILLA SOUP

Be sure to taste your salsa verde to make sure it's to your liking, as that's what brings much of the flavor profile to this soup.

This soup is a great option for using leftovers from the Mojo Shredded Slow Cooker Chicken (page 65). Simply put the leftover shredded chicken in the soup, and lunch is made! If you don't have shredded chicken on hand, you can use a rotisserie chicken. Some stores also have pulled roasted chicken in the deli section.

Total time: 15 minutes | **Makes:** 4 servings

3 cups chicken stock

2 to 3 cups cooked, shredded chicken (from 2 boneless, skinless chicken breast halves or a rotisserie chicken)

1 (15-ounce) can Great Northern beans, drained

1 cup salsa verde

1 teaspoon ground cumin

2 to 4 milliliters water-soluble CBD

1 cup frozen or canned corn or creamed corn

salt and pepper, as needed

6 corn tortillas, cut into ¼-inch-wide strips (6-inch tortillas work best)

¼ cup olive oil

toppings of choice (such as diced avocado, chopped fresh cilantro, shredded cheese, pico de gallo, sour cream, or hemp seeds)

CHICKEN CHILI SOUP

1. In a large stockpot, stir together the chicken stock, shredded chicken, beans, salsa verde, corn, and cumin.

2. Heat over medium high heat until boiling, then cover and reduce heat to medium low.

3. Let simmer for 2 minutes, then add water-soluble CBD and mix well. Cover again and let simmer for another 3 minutes.

4. Taste, and season with salt and pepper if needed. Serve warm with tortilla strips (see below) and your chosen toppings. For added nutritional benefit, sprinkle in hemp seeds.

TORTILLA STRIPS

1. Preheat the oven to 400°F. Dip both sides of the cut tortilla strips in olive oil and sprinkle with salt; arrange on a baking sheet in a single layer. Bake for 8 minutes, or until crisp and lightly browned. Let cool, then serve with the soup.

THE SLOW VERSION

If time allows, you can use raw chicken breasts to make Chicken Chili Tortilla Soup in a slow cooker. Add 2 or 3 raw chicken breast halves along with the chicken stock, salsa, and cumin and cook on low for 6 to 8 hours or on high for 3 to 4 hours. For the last half hour of cooking time, switch to lower heat if on high heat, then shred the chicken and add remaining ingredients, including water-soluble CBD.

QUICK TIP: Great Northern beans are medium-size white beans (slightly larger than navy beans) that are often used for making baked beans. They have a light, nutty flavor that is easily incorporated into stews and soups. I wouldn't recommend adding CBD cooking oil or CBD butter into this recipe—there isn't anything to absorb it (cream, flour, etc.), and you'll be able to see the oil particles as the CBD separates in the broth. Not the worst thing in the world—fat particles are often visible in homemade soups—but because the CBD is "floating," there's not necessarily a way to guarantee how much is in each serving.

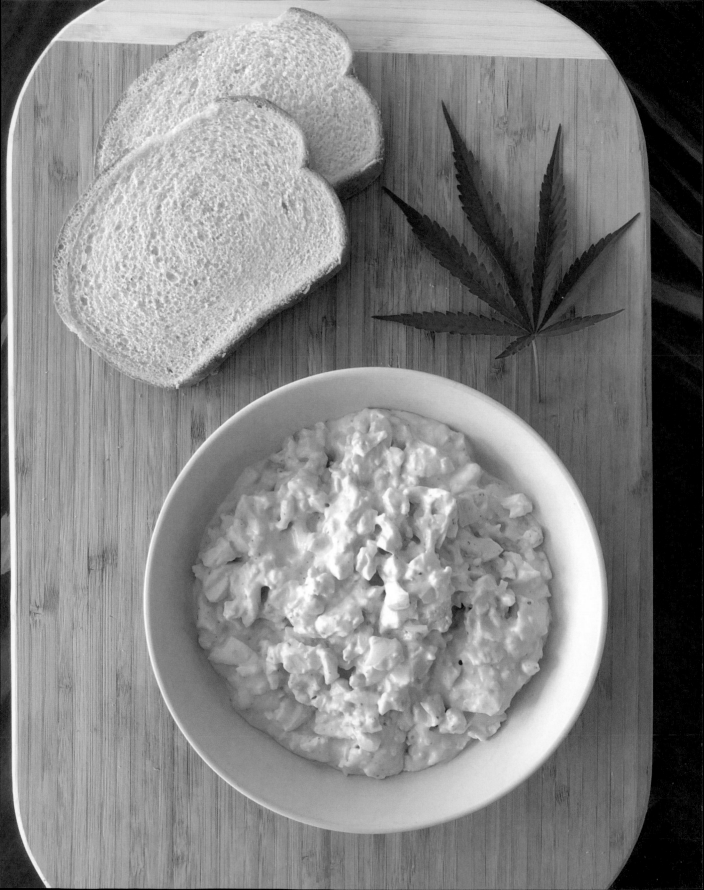

SIMPLY DELICIOUS EGG SALAD

I'm such a fan of egg salad. It's my go-to for a protein-packed lunch or snack. This egg salad is an extra-creamy consistency; the trick is to smash the yolk and mix in the mayonnaise and mustard before adding the egg whites. And thanks to the mustard, this flavorful egg salad is perfect for those who find the average egg salad to be too bland. You can also add your favorite egg salad ingredients, like celery or cooked chunks of potatoes.

Prep and chill time: 30 minutes | **Makes:** filling for 6 sandwiches

12 hard-boiled eggs

¾ cup mayonnaise

3 tablespoons honey Dijon mustard

1½ teaspoons spicy brown mustard

CHOOSE ONE OF THE FOLLOWING CBD OPTIONS
- Instead of ¾ cup of mayonnaise, use ¼ cup of CBD Homemade Mayonnaise (page 108) + ½ cup of unmedicated mayo; or use ¾ cup of Homemade Mayonnaise.
- Add 1 to 2.5 milliliters of water-soluble CBD.

1. Peel the hard-boiled eggs and separate the yolks and the whites into separate bowls.

2. Smash the egg yolks and add the mayonnaise, mustards, and CBD. Mix well.

3. Chop up the egg whites and add to the yolk mixture, combining well. Use immediately or refrigerate to allow the flavors to marry.

4. Enjoy as a sandwich, side dish, appetizer with crackers, or on top of a leafy salad.

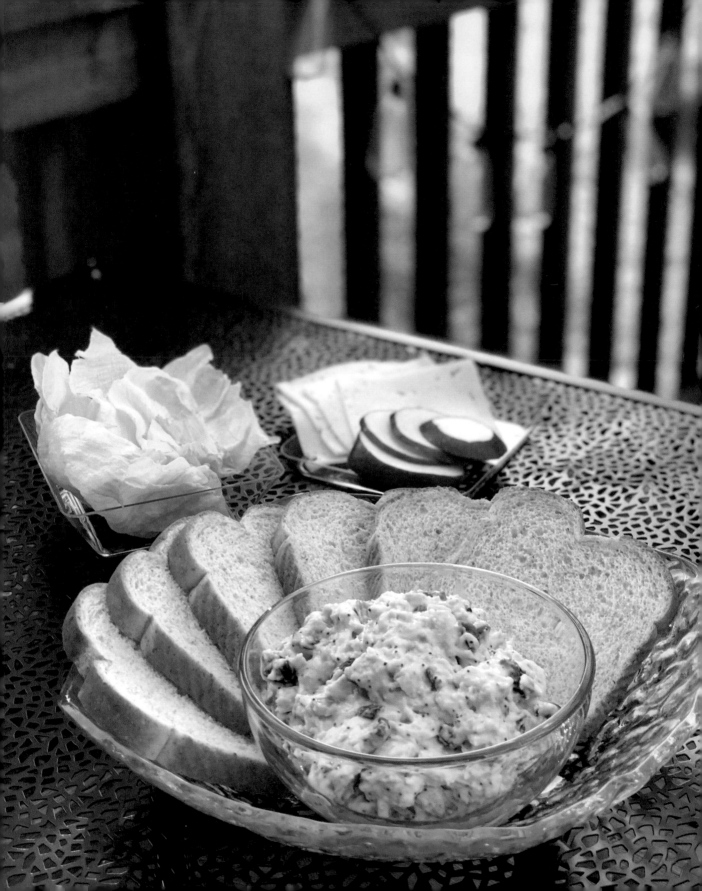

CHICKEN SALAD WITH CRANBERRY PECAN POPPY SEED DRESSING

A rotisserie chicken will give you the amount of shredded meat you need for this salad. Or cook the chicken breasts yourself—season them with 2 teaspoons of salt and add to a large saucepan with 1¾ cups of chicken stock and 5 cups of water. Simmer uncovered, stirring occasionally, until cooked, about 5 minutes. Drain and let cool, then cut into 1-inch pieces for the salad.

Both the chicken and the dressing can be prepared a day ahead and refrigerated. Offer apple slices, cheese, and lettuce as accompaniments.

Total time: 30 minutes | Makes: 4 to 6 servings

DRESSING
½ cup mayonnaise

¼ cup sour cream

¼ cup finely chopped celery

2 tablespoons honey

1 tablespoon Dijon mustard

1 tablespoon poppy seeds

2 tablespoons hemp seeds

salt, to taste

CHICKEN
4 cups chopped cooked chicken breast meat (about 2 boneless, skinless chicken breast halves)

1 cup chopped pecans

½ cup dried cranberries

CHOOSE ONE OF THE FOLLOWING CBD OPTIONS
Instead of ½ cup of mayonnaise, use one of the following:

- ¼ cup CBD Homemade Mayonnaise (page 108) + ¼ cup unmedicated mayo

- ½ cup CBD Homemade Mayonnaise

- ½ cup unmedicated mayo + 4 milliliters water-soluble CBD, combined before adding to other ingredients

1. In a large bowl, combine all the dressing ingredients except the salt. Whisk until well blended, then add salt to taste.

2. Stir in the cooked chicken, pecans, and cranberries and serve as a sandwich filling or as a side salad.

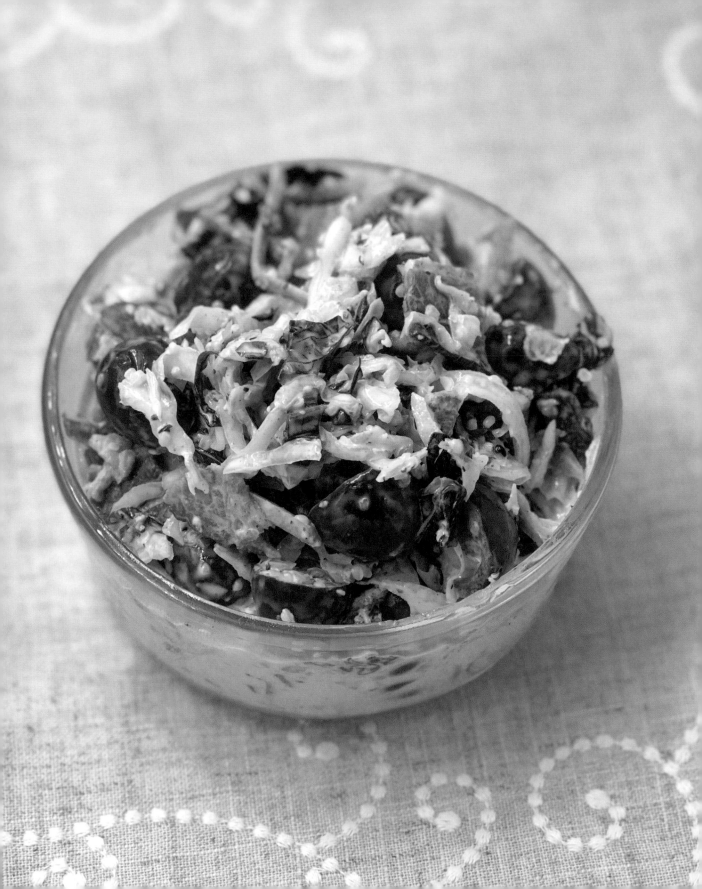

BLT CANNA-SLAW

Using packaged coleslaw mix and carrots saves time and helps cut down on the amount of water that you get with freshly cut and shredded cabbage. In the mood to try something new? Look for bagged coleslaw mixes that include broccoli stems or other vegetables.

Prep and chill time: 1 hour and 10 minutes | **Makes:** 8 servings

8 to 12 slices bacon, cooked

1 cup mayonnaise

¼ cup apple cider vinegar

¼ cup honey or 1 tablespoon sugar

¼ teaspoon dry mustard powder

pinch of salt

6 cups shredded coleslaw mix (prepackaged)

1 cup shredded carrots (prepackaged)

¼ cup chopped fresh basil

1 cup cherry tomatoes, halved

⅓ cup hemp seeds

CHOOSE ONE OF THE FOLLOWING CBD OPTIONS
Instead of the 1 cup of mayonnaise, use one of the following:

• ¼ cup CBD Homemade Mayonnaise (page 108) + ½ cup unmedicated mayo

• ½ cup CBD Homemade Mayonnaise + ½ cup unmedicated mayo

• 4 to 6 milliliters water-soluble CBD added to 1 cup unmedicated mayo

1. Using a blender or a food processor, pulse 4 cooked bacon slices to bits.

2. Roughly chop the rest of the bacon (with a knife) and set aside.

3. In a small bowl, whisk together the mayonnaise, apple cider vinegar, honey or sugar, mustard powder, salt, and CBD until well combined.

4. Add the bacon bits to the dressing and stir to combine.

5. In a large serving bowl, mix together the coleslaw, carrots, basil, tomato halves, hemp seeds, and chopped bacon.

6. Pour the dressing over the coleslaw mix and toss to coat.

7. Refrigerate for an hour before serving to allow the salt to draw out the moisture and marry the flavors. Toss again before serving.

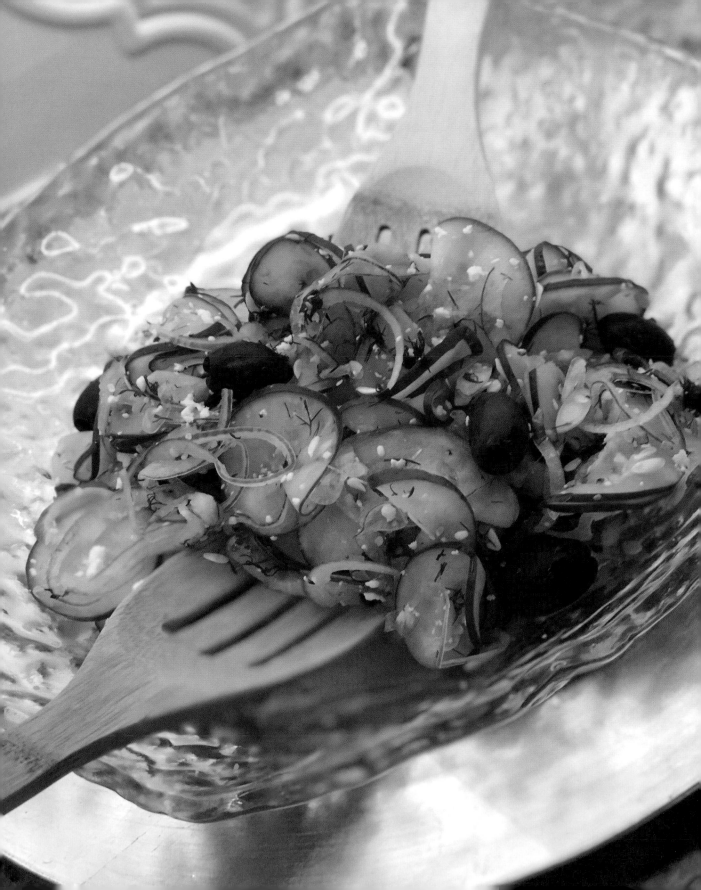

DILL CUCUMBER HEMP SALAD

When making this salad, I use whatever cucumbers are freshest at the store. Usually they have seeds, though cucumbers without seeds or with smaller seeds (English cucumbers) will typically be less watery. If you think your cucumbers are too "wet," you can dry them in the refrigerator for an hour or so before making the salad, as described below. Also pat them with a paper towel to get out excess water. Personally, I don't mind mine a little watery—it helps blend all the flavors.

I generally let these cucumbers pickle for an hour or longer before serving. This is usually the first dish I make when preparing a meal—and it makes a great appetizer. The vinegar and onions really mask the flavor of the CBD, so you can feel free to increase the dosage if needed.

Prep and chill time: 30 minutes plus up to 1 hour chill time | **Makes:** 2 to 4 servings

2 medium cucumbers, thinly sliced (with or without skin)

2 teaspoons salt

2 teaspoons sugar

2 teaspoons red wine vinegar

¼ cup white vinegar

2 to 3 tablespoons hemp seeds

¼ cup chopped fresh dill leaves

1 small red onion, thinly sliced

crumbled feta cheese and pitted kalamata olives, as garnishes (optional)

CHOOSE ONE OF THE FOLLOWING CBD OPTIONS
- **1 to 2 milliliters water-soluble CBD (recommended)**
- **1 tablespoon CBD olive oil or CBD hemp seed oil**

1. Place the sliced cucumbers in a colander set over a bowl. Sprinkle with the salt and sugar, then place in the refrigerator while you prepare the rest of the ingredients. This will help decrease the amount of water in the cucumbers.

2. In a medium bowl, combine the vinegars with the CBD. Then add the hemp seeds.

3. When the hemp seeds are thoroughly coated, add the dill leaves and onion.

4. Remove the cucumbers from the refrigerator and pat dry. Add to the other ingredients, tossing to coat evenly.

5. Refrigerate for at least 20 minutes. Taste to see how pickled the cucumbers are; you can leave them to pickle for an hour or more, depending on taste.

6. When the cucumbers have pickled, toss in crumbled feta cheese and pitted kalamata olives as optional garnishes prior to serving.

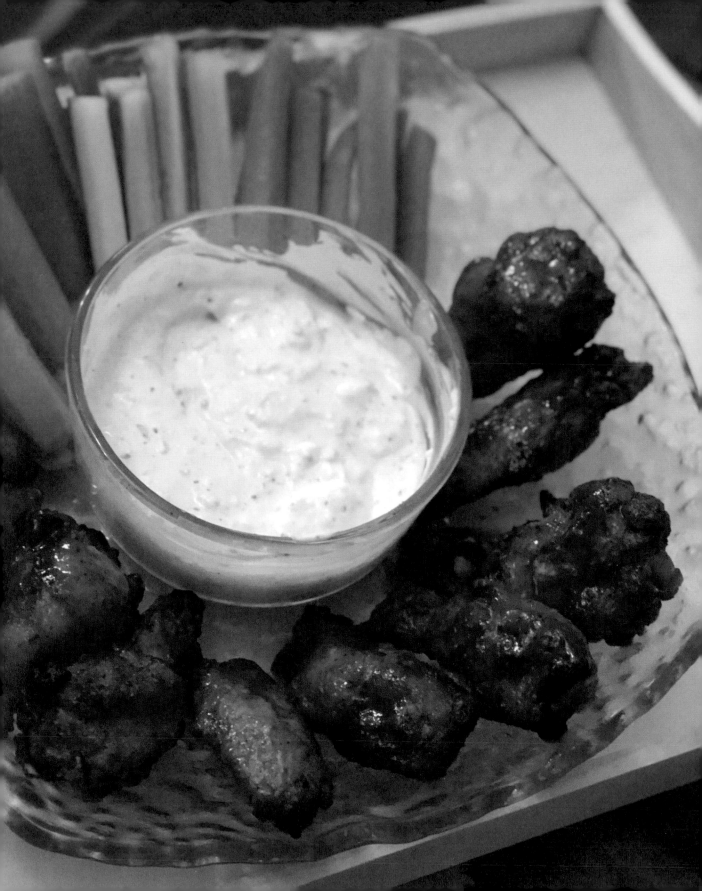

CRISPY BAKED BUFFALO CHICKEN WINGS

How do these wings come out so crispy, as if they'd been deep-fried? Baking powder is the magical ingredient. You won't taste it in the end result—and if you use aluminum-free baking powder, even better. I love my wings extra crispy, so I prefer to eat them plain, with the buffalo sauce and blue cheese dressing on the side for dipping.

Prep and cook time: 1 hour and 10 minutes | **Makes:** 2 or 3 servings

CHICKEN WINGS

4 pounds chicken wings (fresh is better than frozen)

1 tablespoon baking powder

½ teaspoon salt

¼ teaspoon freshly ground pepper

2 teaspoons garlic powder

2 tablespoons vegetable oil, divided

Hemp Blue Cheese Dressing (page 102), carrot strips, and celery strips

BUFFALO SAUCE

½ cup Cholula original hot sauce (or hot sauce of choice)

¼ cup unsalted butter, melted

2 tablespoons honey

CHOOSE ONE OF THE FOLLOWING CBD OPTIONS
- Instead of ¼ cup of unsalted butter, use 2 tablespoons of CBD butter + 2 tablespoons of unmedicated butter.
- Add 1 to 4 milliliters of water-soluble CBD to the buffalo sauce.

1. Adjust an oven rack to the middle position and preheat the oven to 450°F. Line a rimmed baking sheet with aluminum foil and set a heat-proof wire rack inside on the foil. Brush the rack with 1 tablespoon of vegetable oil or spray with cooking spray.

2. Use paper towels to pat the chicken wings, squeezing out as much moisture as possible. If using defrosted wings, they must be totally defrosted and dried.

3. In a medium bowl or large zip-top plastic bag, combine the baking powder, salt, pepper, and garlic powder. Toss the wings in the mixture until all are evenly coated.

4. Arrange the coated wings on the rack in the baking tray, thicker skin side up, leaving about an inch of space between wings. Brush with the remaining vegetable oil.

5. Bake for 30 minutes, then flip the wings over and continue cooking until crisp and golden brown, about 30 minutes longer.

6. While the wings are cooking, make the buffalo sauce. In a small saucepan over low heat, whisk together the hot sauce, melted butter, CBD, and honey. Also, use this time to whip up the Hemp Blue Cheese Dressing, if not previously prepared.

7. When the wings are crispy, remove from the oven and toss them in the buffalo sauce to coat evenly, or serve the sauce on the side as a dip.

8. Serve with the Hemp Blue Cheese Dressing, carrots, and celery.

BAKE-FRIED BIRDS

And if you're wondering, yes, you can use this technique to "bake-fry" Cornish hens, quail, whole chicken, and turkey! For smaller birds up to 4 pounds, I use 2 tablespoons of rotisserie chicken seasoning in place of the garlic. For turkey, you'll have to dial up the amounts and cooking time based on weight, but the formula is 1-part baking powder to 3 or 4 parts salt, plus black pepper to taste. You can include the garlic powder or substitute with rotisserie spices. Sprinkle the spice blend over the thawed and dried turkey. Let the turkey rest in the refrigerator for 12 to 24 hours, and then stick it in the oven. Use a meat thermometer to ensure that the meat is cooked completely. The general rule of thumb is 13 minutes of cooking time for each pound of turkey, but this typically equates to approximately 80 minutes for the breast meat to reach a minimum of 165°F in the thickest part of the thigh. If you press down on the breast plate to flatten the turkey before sticking it on the baking sheet, it cooks faster (no need to flip it over while it cooks). Let rest for 20 minutes before serving.

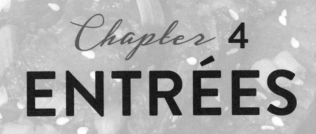

Chapter **4**
ENTRÉES

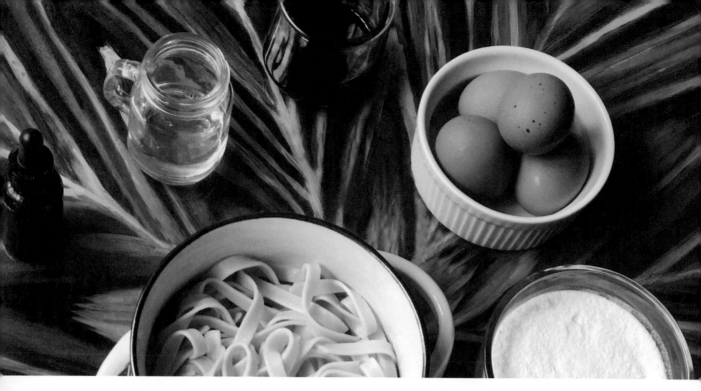

HOMEMADE HEMP PASTA

What I love about making homemade pasta is kneading the dough. It's relaxing and super effective for reducing stress—kind of like making slime with my daughter from glue and contact solution. But kneading homemade pasta is less messy *and* you get to eat something nutritious when you're done!

This pasta takes about 30 minutes to make, start to finish, not including the cooking time (cooking time is approximately 5 minutes).

Total time: 30 minutes | **Makes:** 4 to 6 servings

2½ **cups pasta flour**

4 **eggs**

2½ **tablespoons CBD Rosemary Cooking Oil (page 16), made using olive oil**

2½ **tablespoons hemp seed oil (can be infused with CBD)**

CHOOSE ONE OF THE FOLLOWING CBD OPTIONS
- Instead of CBD olive oil, use unmedicated olive oil + 2 to 4 milliliters of CBD oil or water-soluble CBD, mixed into the oil before adding it to the dough.
- Instead of CBD olive oil and CBD hemp seed oil, use unmedicated oils + CBD oil and/or water-soluble CBD added to both oils (2 milliliters per oil).
- Add CBD oil or water-soluble CBD, as needed, to both oils for a stronger dosage.

1. Mound the flour on a clean surface lined with parchment paper. Make a well in the flour and crack the eggs into it. Use your fingertips to mix in the eggs.

2. Add the oils, mixing with your fingertips.

3. Knead the dough until all the ingredients are well combined, then roll it into a large ball. Cut into 4 equal pieces.

4. Wrap each dough ball in plastic wrap; chill in the refrigerator for 20 minutes.

5. After the dough has chilled, put a large pot of water on the stove to boil. You'll want to cook the pasta soon after you've made it—otherwise it will dry out.

6. Remove each dough ball from the refrigerator and use a rolling pin to flatten the pasta so it can fit into the widest setting of the pasta machine. Roll the dough through the machine; repeat until the consistency is smooth as silk and ready for shaping. Note: the instructions to feed dough through the machine typically come with the machine and are fairly standard: Run the dough through at the widest setting of the pasta machine, then fold and dust the dough and run it through again before adjusting to a thinner setting. Repeat the process and gradually adjust the setting each time until you've reached the thinnest setting (or desired thinness). After pasta runs through the thinnest setting, use the noodle-cutting attachment to shape the pasta; then cut it to desired length. If you don't have a noodle-cutting attachment, shape and cut the pasta by hand.

7. If you don't have a pasta machine, use a rolling pin to flatten the dough and a pizza cutter or knife to cut it into pieces. To stop the dough from sticking to the table or rolling pin, place parchment paper under and on top of the dough. After forming the strips of noodles, dust lightly with flour to avoid them from sticking to each other.

8. Now it's time to cook the homemade pasta immediately by boiling it in salted water for 5 minutes or less, depending on its thickness; it will float when it's cooked al dente. The temperature in the pot shouldn't reach above 325°F. You can use a candy thermometer to keep track of the temperature if you're concerned, but the CBD will be cooking in the water for a very short time.

QUICK TIP: You may notice some oil particles in the water as the pasta cooks. Feel free to save your pasta water to use in other dishes that require water (such as couscous or rice), as it may contain trace amounts of CBD and may also be flavorful with rosemary.

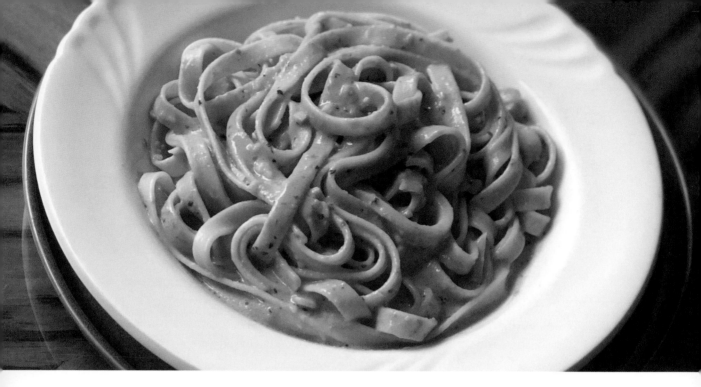

PASTA WITH PINK TOMATO CREAM SAUCE

Pasta with creamy tomato sauce is quick and easy comfort food. In a pinch I've used store-bought grated Parmesan to make this, and it works, but the cheese doesn't melt quite as well. I find that the chicken stock powder gives the sauce a phenomenal amount of flavor, but you can add 1 teaspoon of Italian seasoning and omit the oregano if you feel it needs a little more complexity.

If you want more CBD, you can add water-soluble CBD in Step 6 when you add the pepper. Just be sure to mix the thickened sauce really well.

Total time: 20 minutes | **Makes:** 4 to 6 servings

Homemade Hemp Pasta (page 54), or dried fettuccine or other pasta of choice, enough to make 6 servings

2 tablespoons butter

3 cloves garlic, minced

1 teaspoon onion powder

1 (8-ounce) can tomato sauce (tomato purée)

¾ cup heavy cream

½ cup milk

¾ cup freshly grated Parmesan cheese, plus more for serving

1 teaspoon dried oregano

1 teaspoon chicken or vegetable stock powder (or 1 ground-up bouillon cube)

salt and freshly ground pepper

CHOOSE ONE OF THE FOLLOWING CBD OPTIONS
- 1 to 2 tablespoons CBD rosemary olive oil, or other CBD cooking oil
- 1 to 2 tablespoons CBD butter
- 2 to 4 milliliters water-soluble CBD

1. Boil salted water and cook your pasta for the required time (check package directions if not homemade), minus 2 minutes to ensure that it's al dente. (If you're cooking with the homemade hemp pasta, cook the pasta last; it should only take 4 to 5 minutes.)

2. While the pasta is cooking, melt the butter in a large skillet over medium heat; add the garlic and onion powder and stir. Let simmer for 2 minutes, stirring occasionally.

3. If you're using CBD butter or CBD cooking oil, add the CBD, remove the pan from the heat, and rotate it for a minute or so to let the CBD coat the bottom of the pan.

4. Return the pan to the heat and add the tomato sauce, cream, milk, cheese, oregano, and stock powder. Stir until the cheese is melted.

5. Simmer for 2 minutes, turning the heat up if necessary.

6. Add salt and pepper to taste and lower the heat. Add water-soluble CBD (or additional doses of CBD) and stir well.

7. The pasta should now be cooked; strain it in a colander, scooping out a cup of the cooking water to set aside.

8. Add the pasta to the sauce and toss for a minute or so, until the sauce thickens and clings to the pasta. If necessary, add some of the pasta water to thin the sauce.

9. Serve immediately, passing additional Parmesan to sprinkle on top.

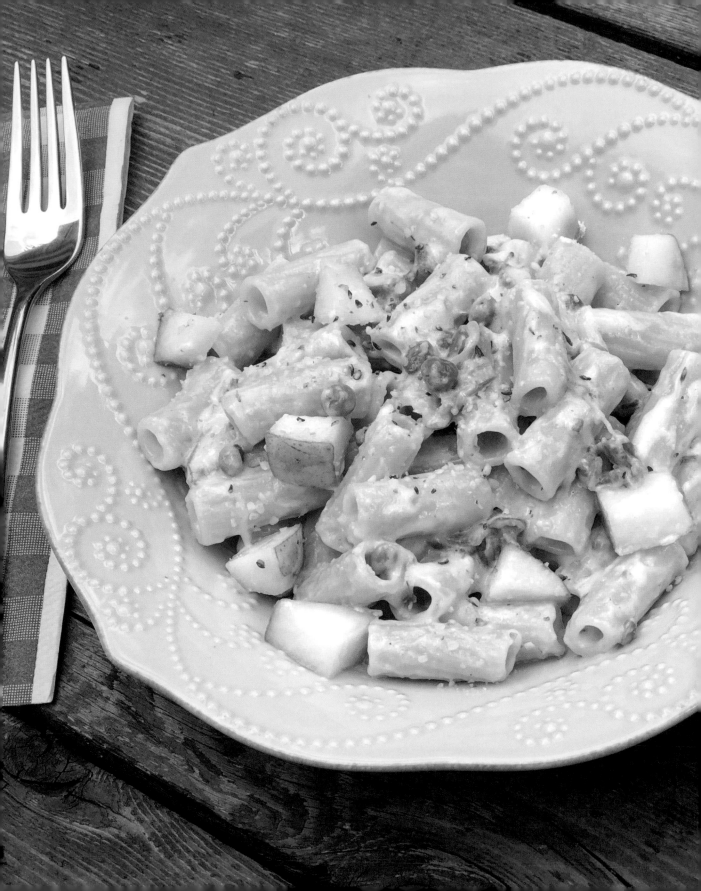

GORGONZOLA ALFREDO PEAR AND PROSCIUTTO PASTA

Sweet pear, salty prosciutto, and tangy Gorgonzola cheese make a winning combination. If you have extra Gorgonzola, you can make Hemp Blue Cheese Dressing (page 102) and pair your pasta with a salad.

Prep and cook time: 25 minutes | **Makes:** 4 servings

8 ounces Homemade Hemp Pasta (page 54) or 8 ounces dried pasta (penne or rigatoni works best)

2 tablespoons unsalted butter

½ cup grated Parmesan cheese, plus more for topping the cooked pasta

1 tablespoon chopped fresh thyme

3 tablespoons crumbled Gorgonzola cheese

½ cup heavy cream

¼ cup frozen peas (petite baby peas work best)

1 large pear, cubed

¼ cup chopped prosciutto

hemp seeds, salt, and pepper, for seasoning and garnish

CHOOSE ONE OF THE FOLLOWING CBD OPTIONS
- Instead of 2 tablespoons of butter, use 1 tablespoon of CBD butter + 1 tablespoon of unmedicated butter.
- Instead of 2 tablespoons of butter, use 2 tablespoons of CBD butter.
- Add 2 to 4 milliliters of water-soluble CBD in Step 3.

1. In a large pot, bring lightly salted water to a boil. Add the pasta and cook until tender yet still firm to the bite, about 11 minutes (check package directions). If using homemade pasta, the cooking time will be less. Drain using a colander.

2. Return the drained pasta to the pot; add the butter/CBD butter, Parmesan, thyme, and Gorgonzola. Place over medium heat and stir just until the cheese is completely melted.

3. Mix the cream and water-soluble CBD, if using, until well combined. Pour onto the pasta and stir.

4. Add the peas and stir until well mixed.

5. Remove from heat and fold in the chopped pear and prosciutto.

6. To serve, top with a sprinkling of hemp seeds. Season with additional Parmesan and add salt and pepper, if needed.

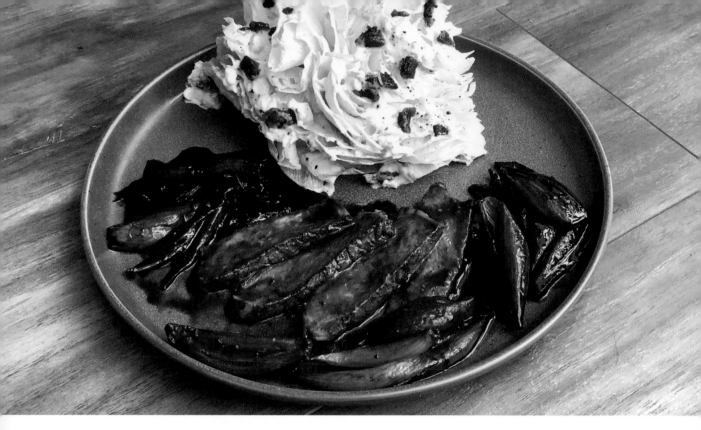

BALSAMIC-GLAZED PORK STEAK

This balsamic vinegar glaze with caramelized shallots is a mouthwatering way to showcase pork steaks. Be sure to choose a balsamic vinegar that you really like, since it's the main ingredient in the sauce. The Hemp Blue Cheese Dressing adds extra sweet and sour notes. This recipe also works with beef steaks and other cuts of pork, following the same process.

You can put the CBD in just the Hemp Blue Cheese Dressing (not in the balsamic glaze) to decrease the overall dosage. If you don't have water-soluble CBD, you can use 1 to 3 tablespoons of softened CBD butter in Step 9. Add a tablespoon at a time until each is fully melted and combined; the resulting glaze will be more of a balsamic butter sauce in consistency.

Total time: 25 minutes | **Makes:** 2 servings

Hemp Blue Cheese Dressing (page 102)

2 pork blade steaks (about 2 pounds total)

salt and freshly ground black pepper

2 tablespoons cooking oil

6 shallots, peeled and quartered, root ends left intact

⅔ cup balsamic vinegar

1½ teaspoons sugar

2 milliliters water-soluble CBD

1. Prepare the Hemp Blue Cheese Dressing; refrigerate to chill.

2. Use a paper towel to pat the steaks dry. Sprinkle on ½ teaspoon salt and ¼ teaspoon pepper.

3. Heat the oil in a 12-inch heavy skillet over moderately high heat until hot but not smoking.

4. Cook the pork steaks (separately, if necessary) with the shallots, turning over once and stirring the shallots occasionally, until the steaks are browned on both sides and the shallots are golden brown and tender, about 5 minutes per side.

5. Use tongs to transfer the steaks to a plate, leaving the shallots in the skillet.

6. Add the balsamic vinegar, sugar, ½ teaspoon salt, and ¼ teaspoon pepper to the skillet and cook, stirring, until the sugar is dissolved and the liquid has thickened slightly, about a minute.

7. Reduce the heat to medium low and return the steaks to the skillet with any juices that have accumulated on the plate, turning them 2 or 3 times to coat with the sauce.

8. Cook, turning once, until cooked to your liking, about 3 minutes or less (if not already cooked as you prefer them, with an internal temperature of 145°F).

9. Transfer the pork steaks to a platter and boil the sauce in the skillet until thickened and syrupy, 1 to 2 minutes. Remove from heat and stir in the CBD.

10. Pour the sauce over the meat. Serve with the Hemp Blue Cheese Dressing.

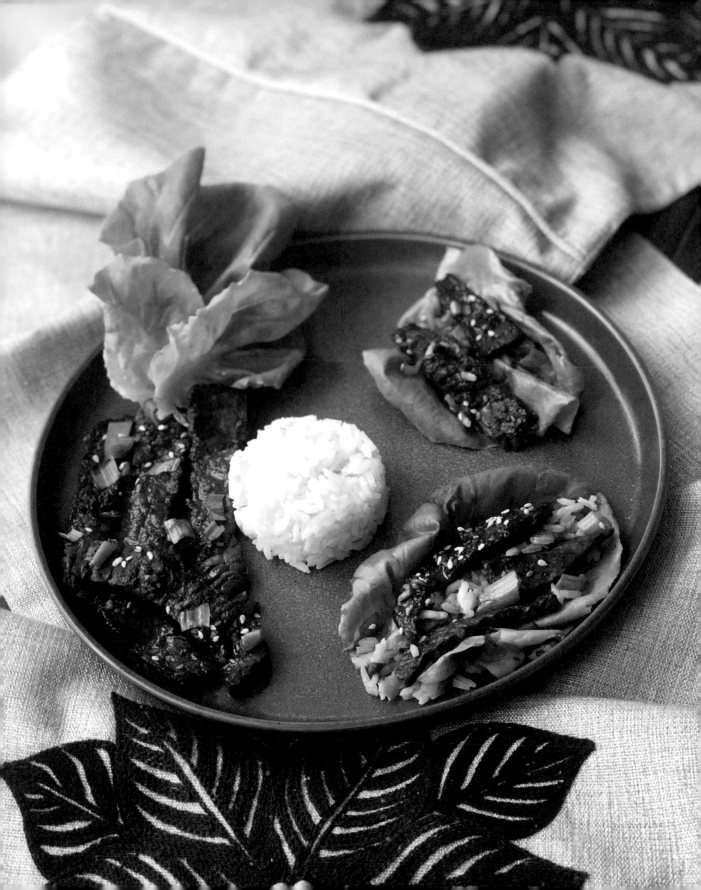

MARINATED BEEF LETTUCE WRAPS WITH COCONUT RICE

Korean-style barbecued beef, or bulgogi, is the inspiration for these tasty lettuce wraps. If your rice isn't soft enough after 20 minutes, or if there's still liquid in the pan or the rice seems soggy, turn the heat up to medium low and cook, covered, until the liquid is absorbed. Or if the rice cooks faster than expected or sticks to the bottom of the pan, add a little water, reduce to lowest heat, cover, and wait for a few minutes for the water to be absorbed.

Total time: 30 minutes | **Makes:** 4 servings

MARINATED BEEF

¼ cup soy sauce

1 tablespoon honey

2 teaspoons sesame oil

1 bunch scallions minced (white and green parts separated)

1 tablespoon minced garlic

1 tablespoon minced fresh ginger

3 tablespoons toasted sesame seeds, divided

1-pound flank steak or London broil, cut across the grain in very thin slices (about ⅛ inch thick)

1 tablespoon vegetable oil

4 milliliters water-soluble CBD

hemp seeds, for garnish (optional)

Boston or other soft-leaf lettuce, for serving; for larger wraps, use a lettuce with a longer leaf, such as iceberg or romaine

COCONUT RICE

1 (14-ounce) can unsweetened condensed coconut milk

1½ cups water

1 tablespoon sugar (optional; I like mine without the added sugar)

2 teaspoons salt

2 cups white rice (jasmine or long-grain)

1 tablespoon CBD coconut oil

sweetened shredded coconut, for garnish

CHOOSE ONE OF THE FOLLOWING CBD OPTIONS
- Instead of water-soluble CBD, use 1 tablespoon of CBD butter in the marinade.
- Instead of CBD coconut oil, use 1 tablespoon of CBD butter in the rice.
- Add 1 tablespoon of CBD butter to the rice in Step 7.

1. In a medium bowl, stir together the soy sauce, honey, sesame oil, white parts of scallions, garlic, ginger, and 2 tablespoons of sesame seeds until well combined. Add the sliced steak and marinate for 15 minutes or refrigerate for 30 minutes or longer.

2. While the steak is marinating, prepare the rice. In a medium saucepan, combine the coconut milk, water, sugar, and salt. Stir until the ingredients are well combined and the sugar is dissolved, then stir in the rice. Bring to a boil over medium heat. Reduce heat, add CBD, cover, and simmer for 18 to 20 minutes.

3. While the rice is cooking, heat the vegetable oil in a 12-inch skillet over high heat until just smoking. Add the steak pieces in a single layer and cook, turning occasionally, until browned on both sides, about 5 minutes total for each batch. Transfer cooked steak pieces to a warm plate or cover to keep warm while the rest of the steak is cooked.

4. Over low to medium heat, add the remaining soy sauce marinade to the pan juices; stir until well combined.

5. Remove from heat and add CBD, stirring well.

6. Toss the steak in the sauce until fully coated, then transfer to a platter and top with the remaining sesame seeds and the scallion greens. If you wish, add a sprinkling of hemp seeds for extra garnish and nutrition.

7. Remove the cooked rice from the heat and fluff with fork. If you wish, you can mix in additional CBD butter. Sprinkle the rice with shredded coconut and serve with the steak and lettuce.

8. To serve, spoon several tablespoons of rice and steak into the center of the lettuce leaf, taco-style, and enjoy.

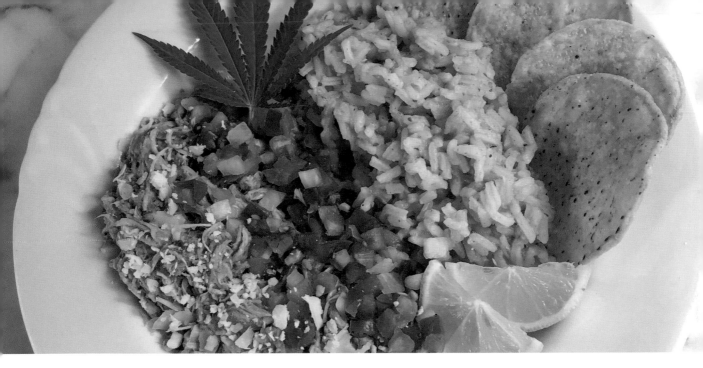

MOJO SHREDDED
SLOW COOKER CHICKEN

This is my kind of recipe—easy to prep in advance. Most slow cookers have a low heat setting of 200°F and a high heat setting of 300°F, so either option will keep the CBD safe. Save the leftover shredded chicken to put into Chicken Chili Tortilla Soup (page 40).

Prep and cook time: about 2½ hours to 5 hours, depending on heat setting |
Makes: up to 6 servings

1 cup orange juice (from 2 or 3 oranges)

¼ cup lemon juice (from 2 or 3 lemons)

½ cup lime juice (from 3 or 4 limes)

1 teaspoon salt

½ teaspoon pepper

1 tablespoon apple cider vinegar

3 tablespoons chopped fresh cilantro, or more as needed

1½ teaspoons ground cumin

2 tablespoons minced garlic

1 tablespoon olive oil

1 teaspoon dried oregano

1 tablespoon minced fresh jalapeño pepper, seeds removed

1½ pounds boneless, skinless chicken breast

6 milliliters water-soluble CBD or 3 tablespoons CBD olive oil

cooked rice, for serving

toppings of choice, such as cheese, pico de gallo, cilantro, and sliced avocado

1. In a food processor or blender, combine all the marinade ingredients (orange juice through jalapeño) and process until well blended.

2. If time permits, pour the marinade into a resealable plastic bag and add the chicken; marinate for 1 hour or more in the refrigerator. If there's not time for that, move on to Step 3.

3. Transfer the marinade and the chicken to the slow cooker. Cover and cook for 2½ hours on high or for 5 hours on low.

4. Once cooked, remove the chicken from the slow cooker and shred, using a pair of forks or knives.

5. Add the CBD to the marinade in the slow cooker and mix well. Return the shredded chicken to the sauce and stir until well combined. Add additional cilantro if needed for flavor.

6. Serve with rice and your chosen toppings, pouring any leftover marinade over the rice and chicken.

SLOW COOKER CARNE ASADA

This marinade is also perfect for slow cooker carne asada or carnitas (pulled pork). Simply swap out the chicken for 1½ to 2 pounds flank or skirt steak or 2 pounds pork shoulder and shred the meat the same way you'd shred the chicken. If you have tortillas and cheese on hand, get ready to make enchiladas for dinner!

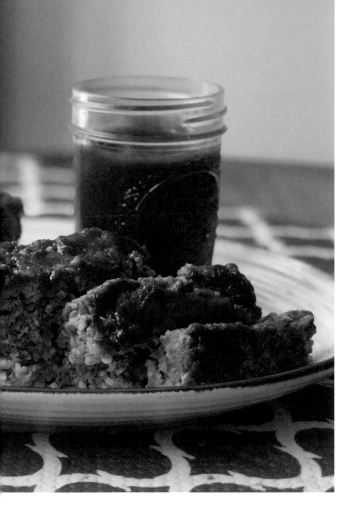

BBQ SMOTHERED MEATLOAF

On the busiest of days, planning dinner can just be completely out of the question. Aside from the CBD, salt and pepper, this recipe calls for only six ingredients.

Prep and cook time: 1 hour and 10 minutes | **Makes:** 5 or 6 servings

1 pound ground beef

1 egg, lightly beaten

1 (8-ounce) can diced tomatoes, drained

½ cup quick-cooking oats, breadcrumbs, or panko breadcrumbs

½ cup minced onion

½ cup minced bell pepper

1¼ teaspoons salt

¼ teaspoon freshly ground black pepper

2 to 3 tablespoons CBD Saint Louis–Style BBQ Sauce (page 115), plus more for serving

1. Preheat the oven to 375°F.

2. In a large bowl, mix together all the ingredients except the BBQ sauce. Stir well.

3. Transfer the mixture to a loaf pan and shape into a loaf.

4. Spread 2 to 3 tablespoons CBD Saint Louis–Style BBQ Sauce over the top of the loaf and bake for 1 hour.

5. Remove from the oven and let cool for a few minutes. Cut into slices; top with additional CBD Saint Louis–Style BBQ Sauce on each serving or on the side as a condiment.

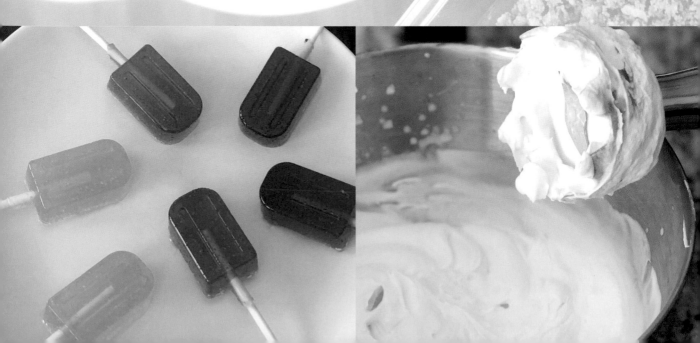

Chapter 5

SWEETS
& DESSERTS

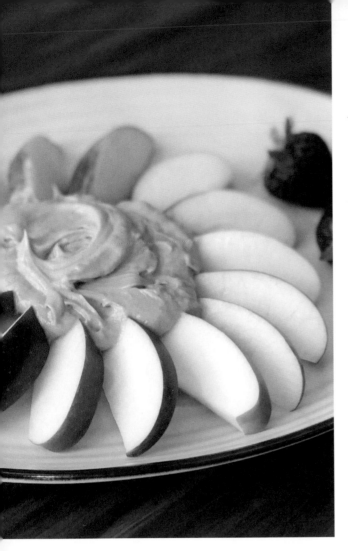

PEANUT BUTTER MOUSSE

The perfect dip for apple slices, this mousse is also incredible on pancakes and as an icing for chocolate cupcakes. Combine it with Graham Cracker Crumble (page 30) for a new take on yogurt parfaits or vanilla ice cream sundaes. Or combine Peanut Butter Mousse, Chocolate Mousse (page 71), Dulce de Leche (page 110), and Graham Cracker Crumble into one dish! If you decide to combine all four in a single dessert, you can opt to scale down the total amount of CBD in each component or make some of these without any CBD.

Prep and chill time: 40 minutes |
Makes: 4 servings

1 cup heavy whipping cream

¼ cup creamy peanut butter

1 teaspoon vanilla extract

4 drops of honey

**1 milliliter water-soluble CBD or
1 tablespoon CBD coconut oil**

1. Combine all the ingredients in a medium bowl and beat with an electric mixer until firm peaks form, about 5 minutes.

2. The mousse will taste great as is, but if you want it to thicken, spoon it into a bowl and refrigerate for 30 minutes before serving.

QUICK TIP: To use Graham Cracker Crumble as a crust for mousse filling, simply press the crumble into the base and sides of a pie plate; you might need up to 4 more tablespoons of butter to make it stick together. Chill in the freezer, and once the crust is frozen, fill evenly with Peanut Butter Mousse or Chocolate Mousse (page 71), or layer one on top of the other. Serve immediately or refrigerate to allow the mousse to stiffen.

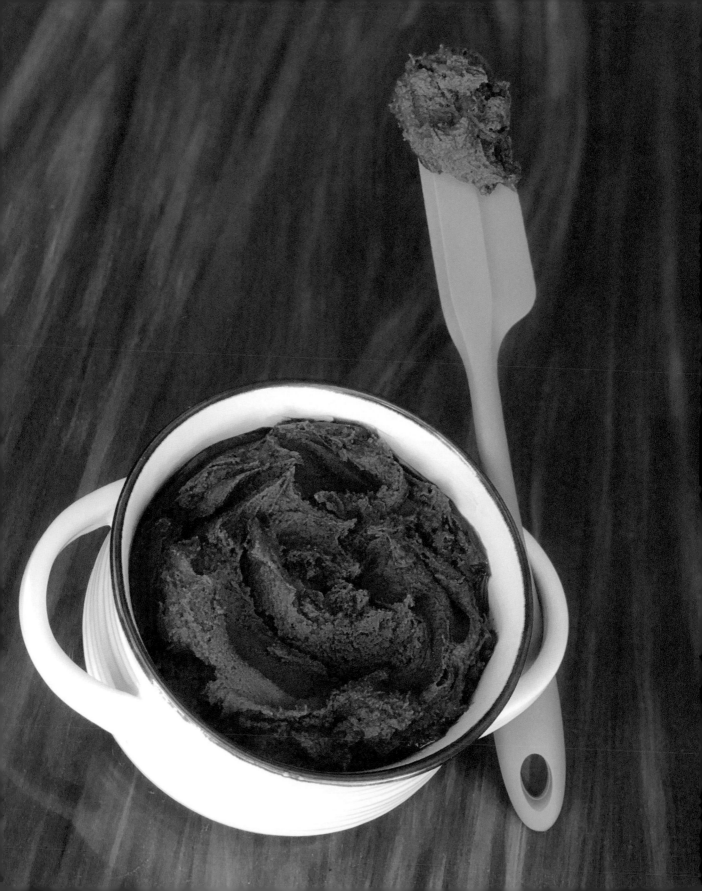

CHOCOLATE MOUSSE

Make sure the dark chocolate you use for this mousse has at least 60% cacao content. I often use bags of chocolate morsels and put them in a food processor before warming them in the microwave with the butter. That helps to melt the chocolate more quickly, and the butter is in the microwave for less time.

Experiment to find your preferred combination of milk and dark chocolate. To make a rich mousse similar to a tart, use all dark chocolate; sprinkle sea salt on top to serve. I've also made this using 2 ounces of milk chocolate and 10 ounces of dark chocolate. As long as there are 12 ounces of chocolate total, you'll have a creamy mouse that's perfect to eat by itself or with fruits such as raspberries and strawberries.

If you have some Graham Cracker Crumble you can sprinkle it on top of the mousse or layer the two with yogurt to make a parfait. Or use the Graham Cracker Crumble as a pie crust for the mousse. Simply fill a frozen crumble crust with the mousse—or layer Chocolate Mousse and Peanut Butter Mousse (page 69). Serve immediately, or chill in the refrigerator to let the mousse stiffen.

Total time: 30 minutes | **Makes:** 6 servings

4 ounces milk chocolate

8 ounces dark chocolate (at least 60% cacao)

1 cup (2 sticks) butter

5 egg yolks

5 egg whites

¼ cup sugar

1¼ cups heavy cream

CHOOSE ONE OF THE FOLLOWING CBD OPTIONS
Instead of 1 cup of regular butter, use one of the following:

- **¼ cup CBD butter + ¾ cup unmedicated butter**
- **½ cup CBD butter + ½ cup unmedicated butter**

---

1. Melt the chocolate with the butter in the microwave or melt on the stovetop in a small saucepan over low heat, stirring every 30 seconds until smooth.

2. Let cool slightly, then stir in the egg yolks, one at a time.

3. In a separate bowl, beat the egg whites with an electric mixer until stiff peaks form. Add the sugar and beat until stiff and white.

4. Carefully stir the egg-white mixture into the chocolate mixture. Let cool in the refrigerator.

5. Whip the heavy cream with an electric mixer, then fold it into the chocolate mixture until well combined.

6. Refrigerate until serving.

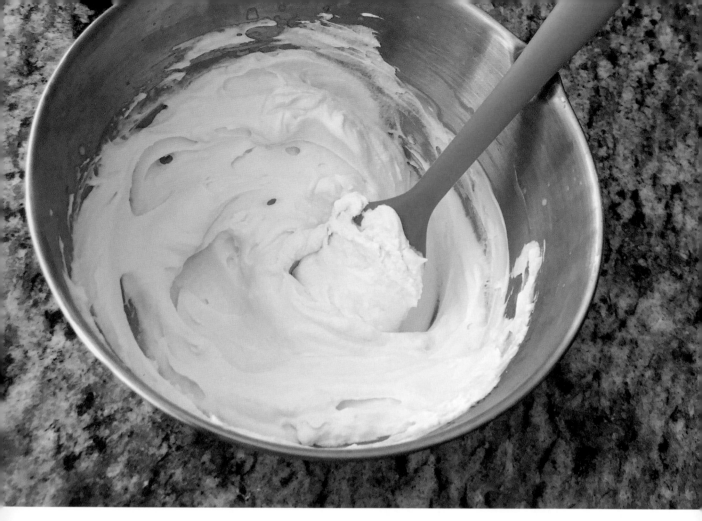

HOMEMADE WHIPPED CREAM

This recipe is easily doubled or tripled. Whipped cream holds its shape for about a day, but if you're looking to keep it in the refrigerator longer, you can use a stabilizer called Whip It (a powder added during the whipping process). Or you can add 1 tablespoon of sifted skim milk powder for every cup of cream and whip until stiff peaks form. Personally, I prefer freezing; frozen whipped cream makes a refreshing treat in the hot summer months, or whenever you need a little CBD.

To make your cream whip faster, use a chilled metal bowl—just place the empty bowl in the freezer until it is cold.

Total time: 5 minutes | **Makes:** 2 cups

1 cup cold heavy cream or heavy whipping cream

2 tablespoons powdered sugar

1 tablespoon CBD Strawberry Syrup (page 113); or use .5 milliliter water-soluble CBD + 1 teaspoon vanilla extract

1. Add all the ingredients to a chilled bowl.

2. Using a hand mixer or an electric mixer with a whisk attachment, whip on medium high speed until medium peaks form, about 3 to 4 minutes. Medium peaks are perfect for pancake toppings. Or you can continue whipping to form stiff peaks, perfect for piping onto desserts.

3. Use immediately, or cover tightly, and refrigerate for up to 24 hours.

TO FREEZE THE WHIPPED CREAM:

1. Spoon the whipped cream into a ¼-cup measuring cup to ensure consistent CBD dosage, then plop onto a parchment-lined baking sheet.

2. Place the filled baking sheet or silicone mold in the freezer.

3. When the cream is frozen solid, place the mounds in a sealable plastic bag and store in the freezer.

4. Use your frozen whipped cream mounds to top hot chocolate, coffee, waffles, or pancakes. When using on top of pie or cake, let the whipped cream thaw for 15 to 20 minutes on the plated dessert before digging in.

QUICK TIP: If you're feeling decorative and have a silicone mold handy, you can use a piping tip to make little swirls in each mound of whipped cream (or spoon the whipped cream into a plastic bag, remove the air, and seal; cut a small hole in one corner and squeeze the cream through the hole to achieve the same effect as a piping tip). Swirl the whipped cream into each mold as evenly as possible to keep the CBD consistent.

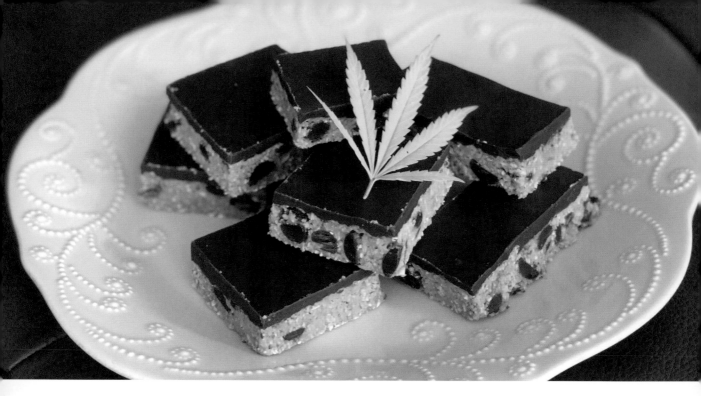

NO-BAKE CHOCOLATE CHIP COOKIE DOUGH BARS

For these cookies, I prefer to put CBD only in the chocolate topping, but if you're looking for a stronger dose you can put CBD butter in the cookie dough as well. You might be able to taste it, but it won't be overpowering. For extra nutrition, add hemp seeds to the oat flour by combining 2 cups of old-fashioned oats with ⅓ cup of hemp seeds in a blender to make a fine flour.

You can use a circular baking pan, and this will look like one giant chocolate chip cookie!

Prep and chill time: 2½ hours | **Makes:** up to 16 servings

COOKIE DOUGH
2⅓ cups old-fashioned oats

½ cup (1 stick) unsalted butter, softened

1 cup packed brown sugar

1 teaspoon vanilla extract

½ cup milk (can be non-dairy)

½ teaspoon salt

1 cup mini chocolate chips

CHOCOLATE GANACHE TOPPING
1½ cups semisweet chocolate chips

2 tablespoons CBD coconut oil

1. Make oat flour by pulsing the oats in a blender or food processor until the texture resembles a fine, powdery flour.

2. In a large mixing bowl, beat the softened butter and brown sugar until well combined.

3. Add the vanilla, milk, salt, and oat flour. Mix until smooth.

4. Fold in the mini chocolate chips until well distributed.

5. Line an 8x8-inch baking pan with parchment or wax paper. Spread the dough evenly in the pan, making sure to get it all the way into the corners. Refrigerate for at least 2 hours, or until firm.

6. To make the top layer, melt the remaining chocolate chips with the CBD coconut oil in a small saucepan over low heat.

7. Spread the topping evenly over the chilled cookie dough. Return the pan to the fridge until the chocolate layer has solidified, about 15 minutes.

8. Cut into 2-inch squares and serve or keep refrigerated.

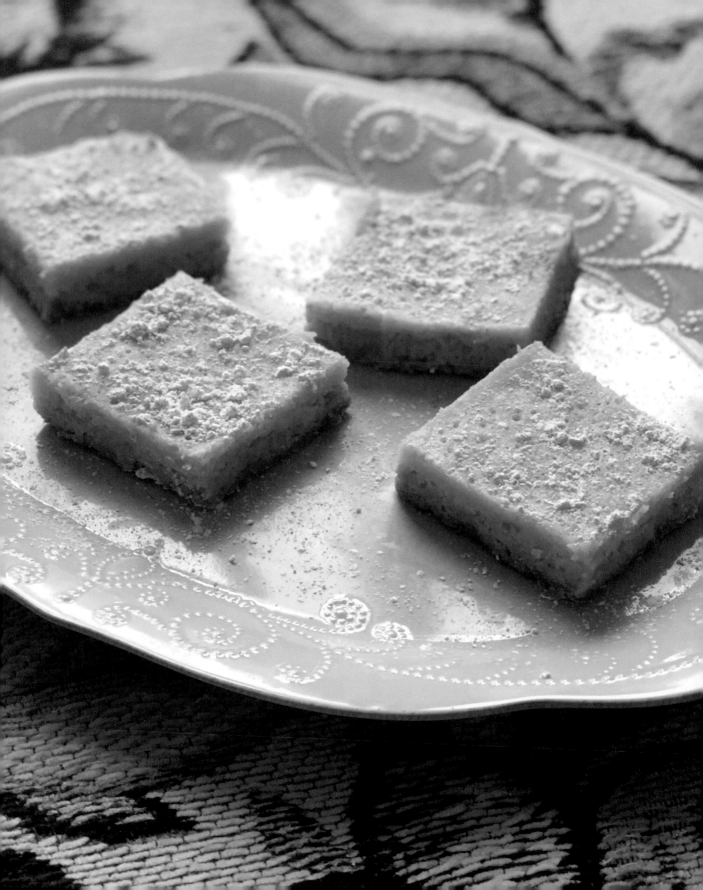

SAINT LOUIS GOOEY BUTTER CAKE

A St. Louis tradition, this classic dessert is addicting! The cake will get a little stickier in consistency once refrigerated, so I typically leave it out for a day or two (if it isn't gobbled up first). It's a crowd-pleaser that can be served with tea and coffee. If you opt to bake the cake without CBD, you can drizzle on some CBD Strawberry Syrup (page 113) or CBD Homemade Whipped Cream (page 72).

Prep time: 10 minutes | **Cook time:** 40 to 45 minutes | **Makes:** 6 to 12 servings
(depending on the size of your sweet tooth)

BOTTOM CRUST

1 (15.25-ounce) box yellow cake mix (any brand, but must be yellow)

½ cup (1 stick) unsalted butter, softened

1 large egg

FILLING LAYER

8 ounces cream cheese, softened

2 cups powdered sugar, plus 2 tablespoons for topping

1 teaspoon vanilla extract

2 large eggs

CHOOSE ONE OF THE FOLLOWING CBD OPTIONS

- Instead of ½ cup of unsalted butter for the crust, use ¼ cup of CBD butter + ¼ cup of unmedicated unsalted butter.
- For the filling, mix 2 teaspoons of water-soluble CBD with the 2 eggs before adding the eggs in with the other ingredients (Step 4).

1. Preheat the oven to 325°F. Spray a 9x13-inch baking dish with cooking spray and set aside.

2. In a mixing bowl, beat the cake mix, butter, and 1 egg with an electric mixer until combined. (The mixture may still be slightly crumbly.)

3. Pour the mixture into a prepared pan and spread it evenly over the bottom. Press down to create an even, slightly firm layer.

4. In a mixing bowl, beat together the cream cheese, powdered sugar, vanilla, and 2 eggs for about 3 to 4 minutes, until well combined.

5. Pour the cream cheese mixture over the crust; use a spatula to spread evenly.

6. Bake for 40 to 45 minutes, until the filling is lightly browned. Remove from the oven and let cool completely or refrigerate. Sprinkle with powdered sugar before serving.

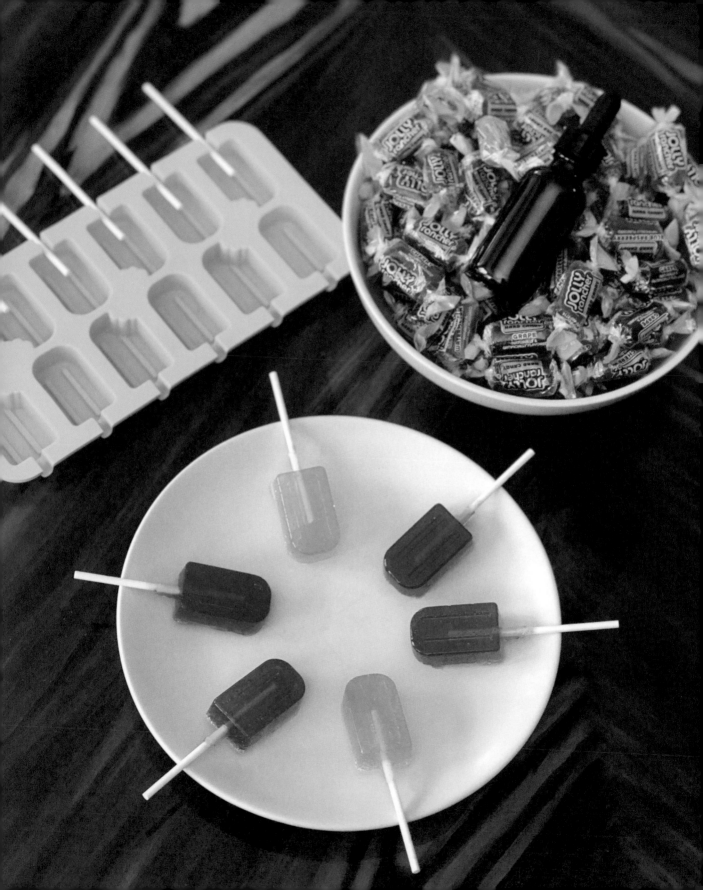

CBD JOLLY RANCHER LOLLIPOPS

I've made lollipops the traditional (hazardous) way—combining sugar, corn syrup, and cream of tartar on the stovetop—and the messy process is one I advise against. In my experience it's a race against time, as the sugar (aka molten lava) doesn't stay pliable long enough to add the CBD. Also, the taste leaves much to be desired even after adding flavored extracts. These Jolly Rancher lollies are much easier and safer to make, and they're much tastier.

You'll need a silicone lollipop mold, and since molds and baking trays can be different thicknesses, be sure to watch your Jolly Ranchers to make sure they melt but don't bubble/boil. If the sugar caramelizes, the color and flavor of the candy changes. It's a good idea to prep all work surfaces and the baking tray with parchment paper in case any candy drips out of the mold.

When you stir in water-soluble CBD, the candy mixture might bubble or fizz a bit—a normal reaction for sugar. Move quickly when mixing in the CBD, as the candy will start to harden as soon as it is removed from the oven. Keeping the mold on the hot tray can buy you some time while you mix in the CBD.

At .25 milliliter, you might taste some of the CBD, since the lollipops are small. If you add more than that, the flavor of the CBD might be overpowering. You could increase the amount of water-soluble CBD by using a flavored CBD or by finding a mold that holds more than 3 candies per lollipop.

Prep and rest time: about 45 minutes | **Makes:** 3 Jolly Ranchers make 1 lollipop

Jolly Rancher candies   **silicone lollipop mold**

.25 milliliter water-soluble CBD per lollipop   **lollipop sticks**

1. Preheat the oven to 350°F.

2. Separate the candies by flavor and place them into the lollipop mold (usually 3 candies per opening).

3. Place the mold on a thin baking sheet and put in the oven for 5 to 10 minutes, or until the candy is melted. If the candy starts to form bubbles, remove it immediately before the sugar starts to caramelize.

4. Remove from the oven and drop .25 milliliter of water-soluble CBD into each candy. Use a lollipop stick to quickly stir, then set a stick into each mold.

5. Once the CBD has been incorporated, transfer the candy to a cooling rack and let it fully harden before unmolding it, about 30 minutes. Or you can let it harden slightly and then refrigerate it to speed up the process.

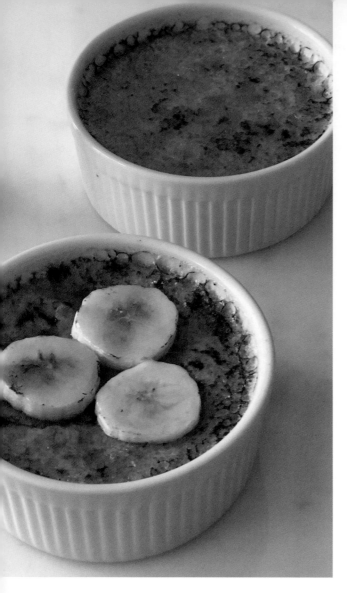

VANILLA PUMPKIN SPICE CRÈME BRÛLÉE

If you don't have ramekins, you can make this dessert in small, decorative bowls, or whatever you have that's ovenproof. If you wish, you can top your custards with fresh berries, caramelized bananas, or CBD Homemade Whipped Cream (page 72).

To make a more traditional crème brûlée, simply leave out the pumpkin pie spice.

Total time: about 4 hours |
Makes: 4 servings

¾ teaspoon vanilla extract

1 tablespoon pumpkin pie spice

2 cups heavy cream

4 large egg yolks

4 milliliters water-soluble CBD

⅓ cup + 2 teaspoons (3 ounces) sugar

pinch of salt

1 to 2 teaspoons of superfine sugar for each custard ramekin

1. Preheat the oven to 300°F. Fill a kettle with water and bring to a boil. Arrange 4 ramekins in a large baking dish, far enough apart that they aren't touching. Set aside.

2. In a medium saucepan, stir together the vanilla, pumpkin pie spice, and heavy cream. Heat over medium heat until simmering but not boiling. Stir occasionally.

3. When the cream is simmering and the ingredients are well combined, remove from the heat and let sit for 5 minutes.

4. Use an electric mixer on medium speed to combine the egg yolks, water-soluble CBD, 3 ounces of sugar, and salt, beating for about 1 minute until light and smooth.

5. Slowly add the cream mixture to the eggs, using the electric mixer to combine.

6. Pour the liquid into the ramekins until evenly distributed. If you notice any cooked egg particles, strain all the liquid through a mesh strainer or cheesecloth. (Eating bits of lumpy egg in creamy custard can be disconcerting.)

7. Pour the boiling water from the kettle into the pan so that it reaches ⅔ of the way up the sides of the ramekins. It's important for the water to be boiling when it enters the pan in order for the custard to cook properly.

8. Bake for 45 to 50 minutes, or until the edges of the custard are set and the centers are slightly jiggly but not liquidy.

9. Carefully remove the pan from the oven and use tongs to transfer the ramekins to a cooling rack. Or set the pan on the cooling rack and wait until the ramekins have cooled enough to move easily. Let the custard come to room temperature, then refrigerate for at least 3 hours, until cool.

10. When ready to serve, evenly sprinkle 1 to 2 teaspoons of superfine sugar onto each custard, then use a kitchen torch to caramelize the sugar. Hold the torch 2 to 3 inches from the surface and slowly move the flame back and forth until the sugar is a deep amber color and bubbly. Let the custard sit for about a minute before breaking a spoon into it.

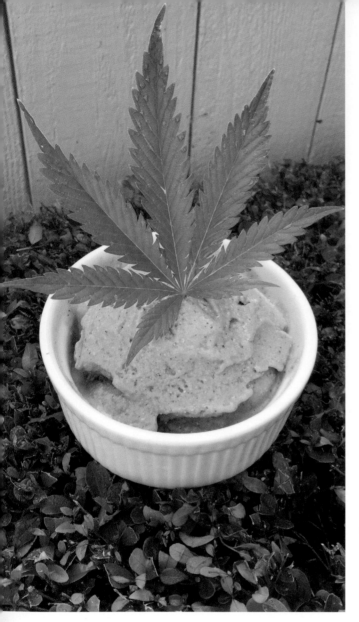

STRAWBERRY HEMP SORBET

If you don't have an ice cream machine, you can pour the strawberry purée onto a rimmed, parchment-lined cookie sheet and freeze until set. Allow it to defrost slightly and then chop the frozen purée into pieces and blend again in a blender or food processor. (Separate into batches, if needed.) Serve immediately or, for the most sorbet-like consistency, freeze on the cookie sheet once more and blend again.

You can also use this recipe to make a strawberry smoothie.

Total time: 10 minutes |
Makes: 1½ quarts

½ cup plus 1 tablespoon hulled hemp seeds (crunchy outer shell removed)

2 pounds strawberries

1¼ cups water

½ teaspoon ground raw vanilla beans or vanilla bean paste

6 pitted dates

1 tablespoon lecithin powder (as a natural emulsifier)

CHOOSE ONE OF THE FOLLOWING CBD OPTIONS
• Add 2 to 3 tablespoons of CBD coconut oil or CBD hemp seed oil.

• Add 6 milliliters of water-soluble CBD.

1. Using a blender, purée all the ingredients together for about 2 minutes.

2. Pour into an ice cream machine and process until the mixture reaches a sorbet consistency.

3. Serve at once, or transfer to another container and store in the freezer.

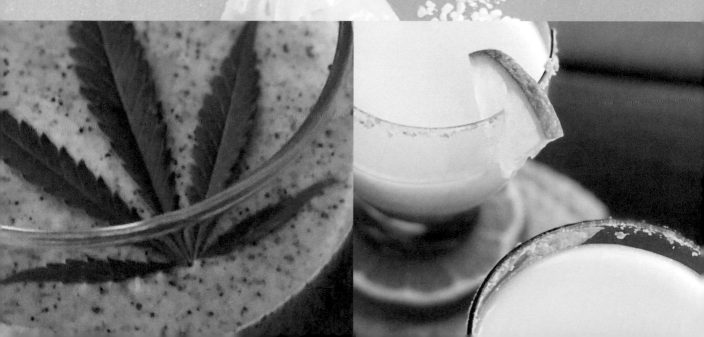

Chapter **6**

HEMP SMOOTHIES
& DRINKS

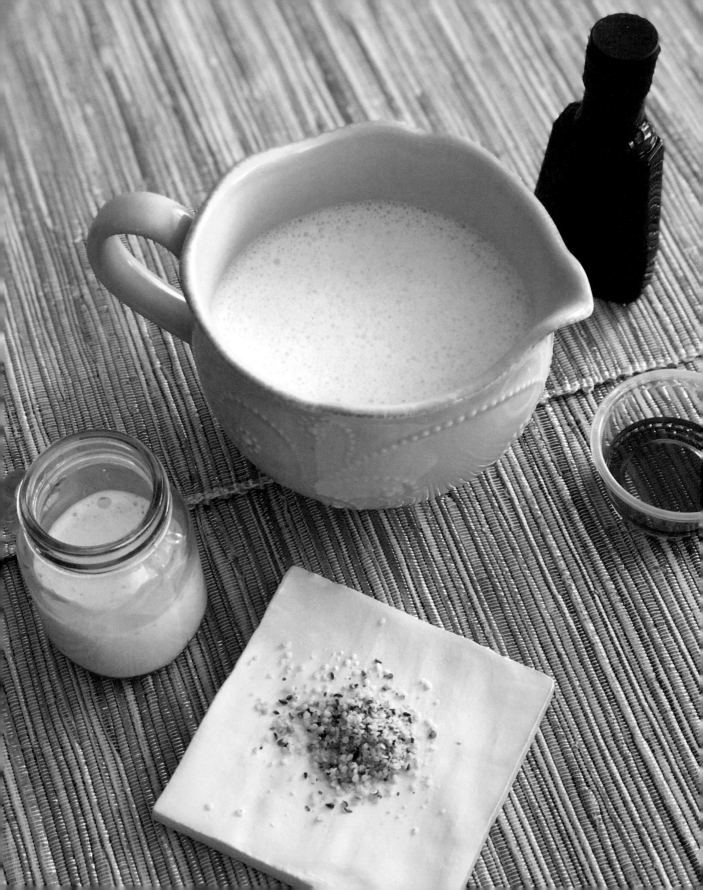

FAST & EASY VEGAN HEMP MILK

Hemp milk has a creamy consistency that is slightly thicker than skim milk and a nutty flavor that is similar to almond milk. This dairy-free milk alternative is refreshing on its own or it can be used as a nutritious base for fruit smoothies. Straining out the seeds (Step 3) is up to your personal preference—I don't mind hemp seeds in my milk, and I feel like it's more nutritious to leave them in. I prefer using hulled hemp seeds (without shells), as I find that they blend much better for a creamy consistency.

If you decide to strain your milk, the seeds that are left on the cheesecloth can be used in oatmeal or in No-Bake Chocolate Chip Cookie Dough Bars (page 74), as they'll still have nutritional value.

Total time: 5 minutes | **Makes:** 2¼ cups

½ cup hemp seeds

2 cups water, divided

½ teaspoon vanilla extract

1 tablespoon maple syrup

CHOOSE ONE OF THE FOLLOWING CBD OPTIONS
- .5 to 1 milliliter water-soluble CBD (recommended)
- 1½ teaspoons CBD hemp seed oil

1. Place the hemp seeds in a blender with 1 cup of water. Blend until smooth and creamy, about 2 minutes.

2. Add the remaining water. Blend for about 2 more minutes.

3. For ultra-creamy milk, strain the hemp milk through cheesecloth to remove all the seed pulp, then pour the liquid back into a blender.

4. Add the vanilla, maple syrup, and CBD and blend. Serve immediately, or chill in the refrigerator. The hemp milk will separate a bit when refrigerated, so it's best to stir it before serving or blend it again for a couple of seconds.

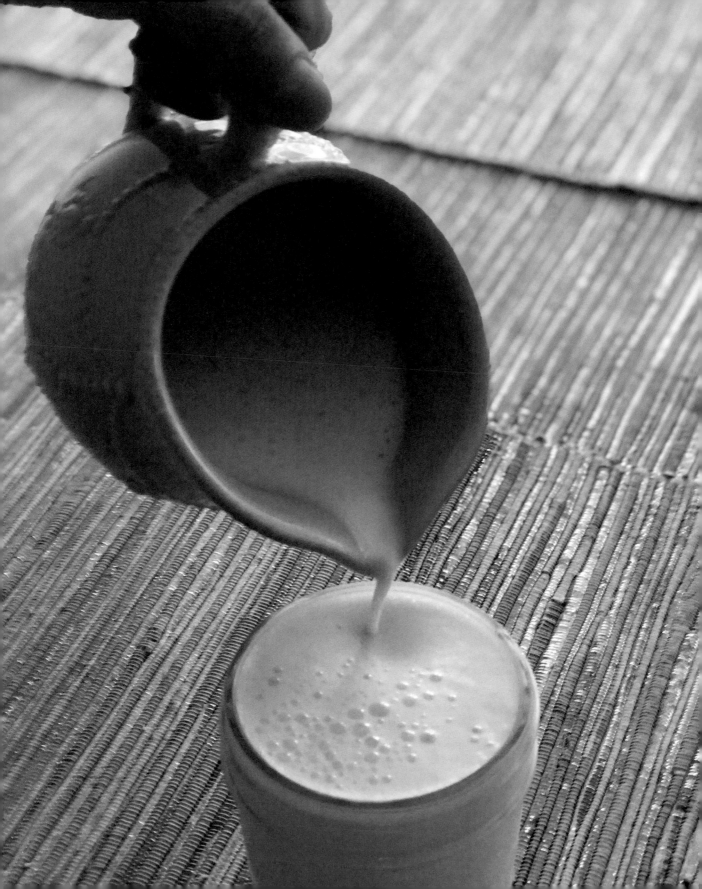

BHANG LASSI–INSPIRED CANNABIS MILK SHAKE

Adding milk is an easy way to increase the already-packed nutritional value of hemp milk. The Bhang Lassi originated in India and is the first known cannabis milkshake. In medicinal lore, it's referenced as a cure for pain; in ancient Hindu religious ceremonies it was used to connect the followers of Shiva to the deity. Today numerous variations are consumed during holy days and festivals, and it's also used as a holistic health aid for fever, pain, stress, sleep problems, and other ailments.

Traditional Bhang Lassi is a labor-intensive drink that requires many ingredients, including raw marijuana buds. Spices and nuts—such as ginger, almonds, cashews, saffron threads, cardamom, anise, nutmeg, garam masala, and fennel seeds—are steeped with raw marijuana and milk to make tea. The process involves several steps of heating, draining, and cannabis-grinding. This is a much simpler version with fewer ingredients. While hemp leaves and hemp flower won't get you high, the raw plant material has antioxidants and anti-inflammatory benefits.

Total time: 15 minutes | **Makes:** 2¼ cups

1 hemp flower and 1 or more hemp leaves, divided

1 cup sweetened vanilla almond milk

1 cup vanilla coconut creamer

1 stick cinnamon or ½ teaspoon ground cinnamon

½ cup hemp seeds

1 cup ice cubes (optional)

CHOOSE ONE OF THE FOLLOWING CBD OPTIONS
- .5 to 1 milliliter water-soluble CBD (recommended)
- 1½ teaspoons CBD coconut oil (if drinking this hot)
- 1 tablespoon softened CBD butter (if drinking this hot)

1. Place the hemp flower in a saucepan with the almond milk, coconut creamer, and cinnamon. Let simmer over low heat for about 5 to 10 minutes; stir occasionally. Remove the cinnamon stick, if used.

2. In a blender, purée the hot milk, hemp leaves, and hemp seeds. Blend until smooth and creamy, about 2 minutes.

3. If the consistency of the hemp particles isn't to your liking, strain the mixture through cheesecloth, then return the liquid to the blender.

4. Add the CBD and blend again until well combined.

5. Serve immediately if you like it hot or add a cup of ice and blend until smooth and thick.

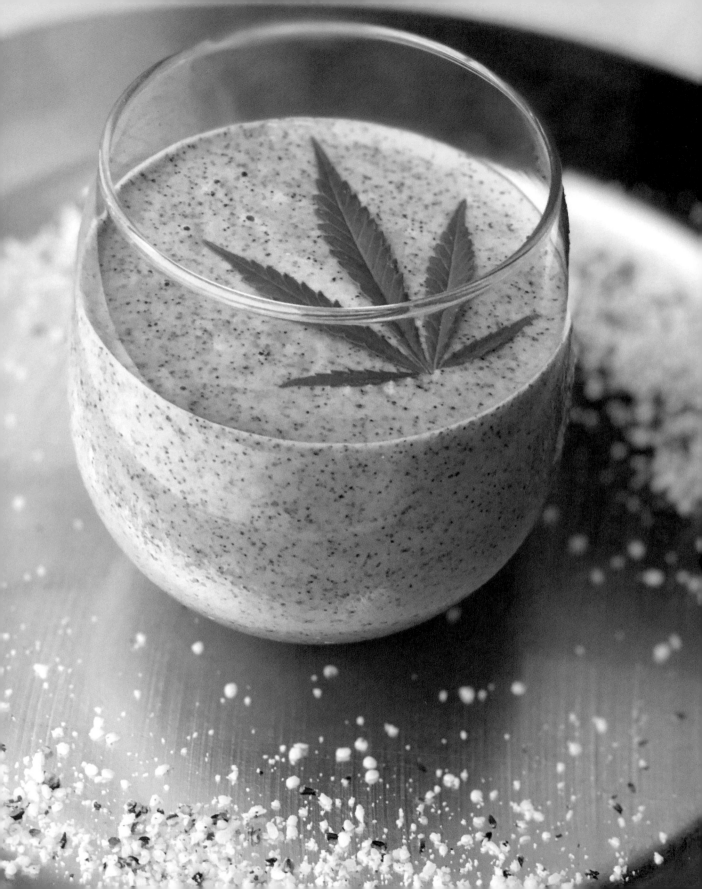

MINT AVOCADO SPINACH SMOOTHIE

Wait...mint? Spinach? *And* avocado? Curiously, yes, these three nutritious yet powerful flavors do taste incredibly refreshing when blended together. The vanilla almond milk and vanilla coconut creamer give just enough sweetness. I personally love making the sweetened hemp milk in this recipe to add to coffee and other drinks. It helps me cut out adding extra sugar and sweeteners.

Total time: 10 minutes | **Makes:** 2 servings

½ cup hemp seeds

1 cup sweetened vanilla almond milk

1 cup vanilla coconut creamer

½ ripe avocado

1 cup spinach leaves

¼ cup fresh mint leaves

4 tablespoons hemp protein powder

1 frozen banana or 1 cup ice cubes

CHOOSE ONE OF THE FOLLOWING CBD OPTIONS
• .5 to 1 milliliter water-soluble CBD

• 1 tablespoon CBD hemp seed oil

1. In a blender or food processor, make sweetened hemp milk by combining the hemp seeds, almond milk, and coconut creamer. Blend for 2 minutes.

2. If you wish, strain through a cheesecloth to remove the hemp seeds, then return the mixture to the blender.

3. Add the CBD, blend for 2 minutes, and then add the remaining ingredients except for the frozen banana or ice. Blend for an additional 2 minutes.

4. Blend frozen banana or cup of ice into smoothie. Serve immediately.

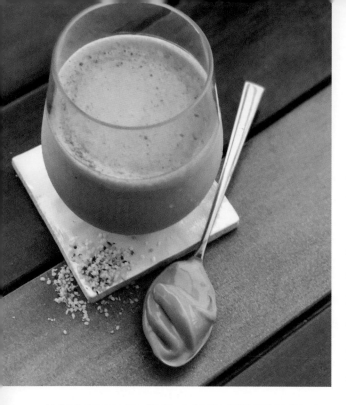

PEANUT BUTTER BANANA SMOOTHIE

For extra energy benefits, you can add a teaspoon of maca powder and a tablespoon of MCT oil when you blend this smoothie.

Total time: 5 minutes | **Makes:** 1 serving

¾ cup Fast & Easy Vegan Hemp Milk (page 85), or more if desired

handful of ice cubes, or more if desired

1 frozen banana

2 tablespoons creamy peanut butter

1 teaspoon unsweetened cocoa powder

CHOOSE ONE OF THE FOLLOWING CBD OPTIONS

• **.5 milliliter water-soluble CBD**

• **1 teaspoon CBD hemp seed oil**

1. Combine the hemp milk in a blender with the rest of the ingredients. Blend until smooth.

2. If desired, add more ice for an icier and thicker consistency or more hemp milk for a thinner consistency before serving the smoothie.

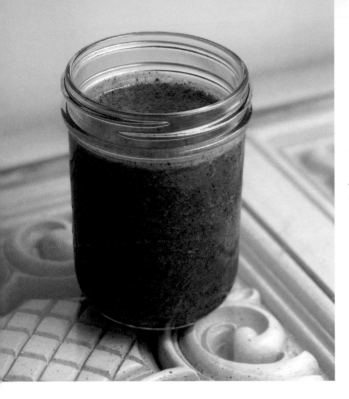

BERRY HEMP SMOOTHIE

Pomegranate and cranberry juice are packed with health benefits, including antioxidants. If this smoothie is a little thick for your liking, add up to ½ cup more juice. For extra hemp nutrients, add 2 to 4 tablespoons of hemp seeds.

I recommend freezing any leftovers as deliciously healthy CBD ice pops, since the ingredients will separate if the smoothie is kept in the refrigerator.

Total time: 5 minutes | **Makes:** 4 or 5 servings

1 cup Fast & Easy Vegan Hemp Milk (page 85), or milk of choice

1 cup flavored yogurt (I like vanilla or one of the flavors of the frozen fruit used in the smoothie)

3 to 4 tablespoons hemp protein powder

1 cup cranberry pomegranate juice or ½ cup *each* cranberry and pomegranate juice

2 cups frozen or fresh berries, preferably blueberries and blackberries

1 cup ice if using fresh berries, or as needed

CHOOSE ONE OF THE FOLLOWING CBD OPTIONS
- 1 to 2 milliliters water-soluble CBD
- 1 tablespoon CBD hemp seed oil

1. In a blender, combine the hemp milk, yogurt, hemp protein powder, and CBD. Mix for 2 minutes.

2. Add the juice and berries and blend for 2 more minutes.

3. Add ice, if necessary, to thicken and make colder, and blend until smooth. Serve immediately.

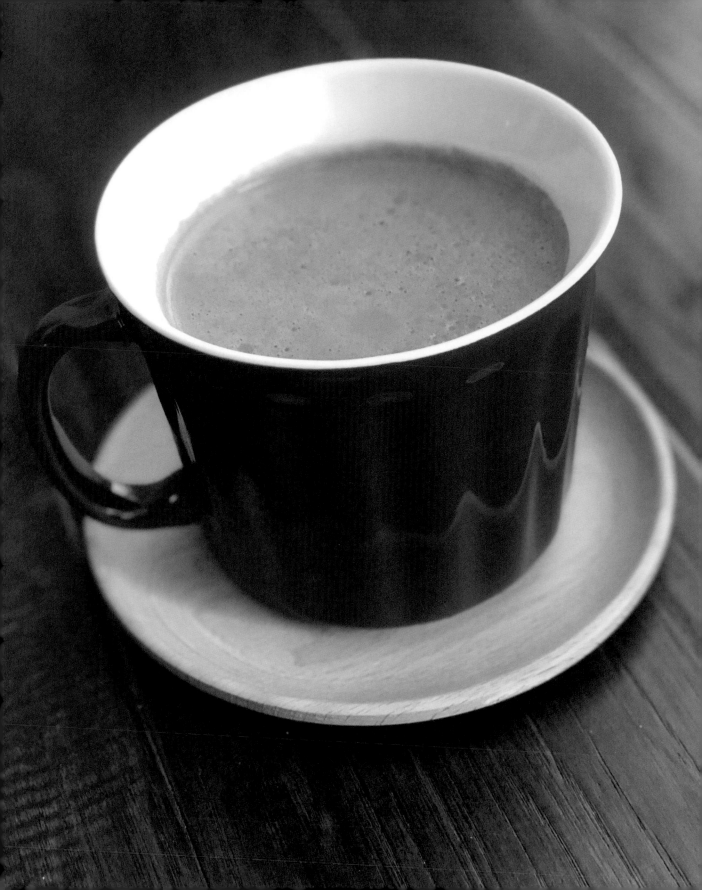

NEXT-LEVEL MOCHA COFFEE

If you've ever heard of bulletproof coffee or keto coffee, this is the CBD version, and it'll really get your brain charged to the next level! MCT oil and maca powder fuel the brain. You can also make this with hot cocoa or hot chai tea instead of coffee.

Pumpkin pie spice can be found in any grocery store with a spice aisle. It's a combination of cinnamon, nutmeg, allspice, ginger, and cloves, so if you don't have pumpkin spice, you can sprinkle in those spices.

While this is delightfully frothy after it's been through the blender, you're going to want to drink it soon, because the MCT oil (and CBD oil/butter) will separate if it's left out for long. For a less bitter taste, use the sweetened hemp milk (hemp seeds, sweetened almond milk, and coconut creamer) in Step 1 of the Mint Avocado Spinach Smoothie recipe (page 89) instead of the Fast & Easy Vegan Hemp Milk.

Total time: 10 minutes | **Makes:** 1 or 2 servings

2 cups hot coffee

1 tablespoon MCT oil

1 teaspoon maca powder

1 teaspoon unsweetened cocoa powder

¼ teaspoon vanilla

¼ teaspoon pumpkin pie spice

¼ cup Fast & Easy Vegan Hemp Milk (page 85), or more, if desired

CHOOSE ONE OF THE FOLLOWING CBD OPTIONS
- **.5 to 1 milliliter water-soluble CBD (recommended)**
- **1½ teaspoons CBD coconut oil (if drinking this hot)**
- **1½ teaspoons softened CBD butter (if drinking this hot)**

1. Combine all the ingredients in a blender and blend for 1 to 2 minutes.

2. Enjoy immediately.

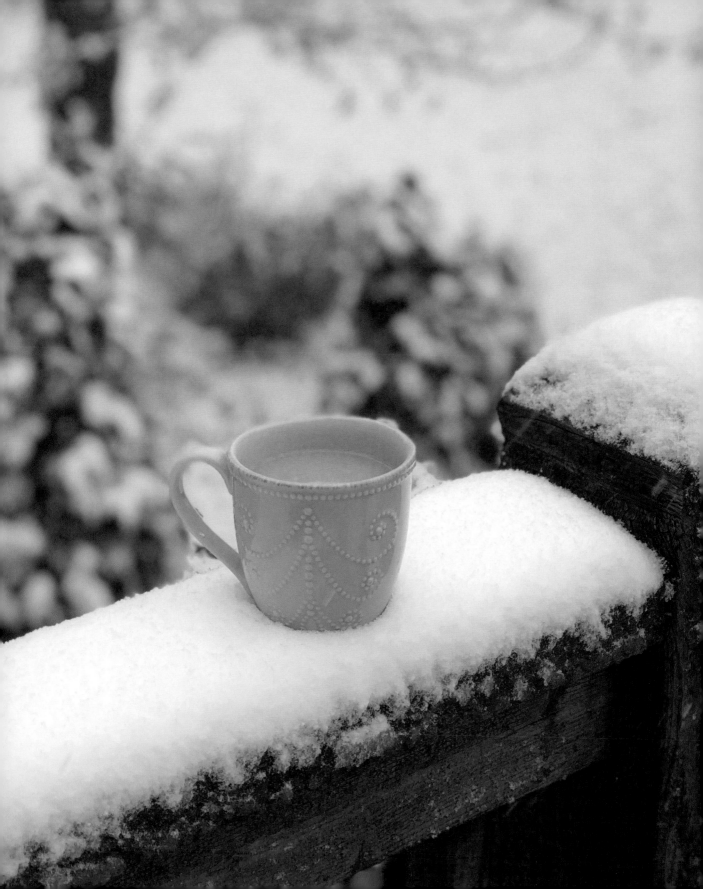

HAZELNUT HOT COCOA WITH BAILEY'S IRISH CREAM

I enjoy combining this hot cocoa with Next-Level Mocha Coffee (page 93) for a café mocha twist. It also tastes amazing as a cold, boozy milkshake. Simply follow the instructions below, then pulse in a blender with 1 cup of ice.

Total time: 10 minutes | **Makes:** 1 serving

1 cup milk (chocolate milk, vanilla almond milk, hemp milk, whole milk, or any kind)

2 tablespoons Nutella

¼ cup Baileys Irish Cream

Homemade Whipped Cream (page 72), for serving

CHOOSE ONE OF THE FOLLOWING CBD OPTIONS

- **.5 milliliter water-soluble CBD (recommended)**
- **1½ teaspoons CBD coconut oil (if drinking this hot)**
- **1½ teaspoons softened CBD butter (if drinking this hot)**

1. Heat the milk in a saucepan over medium high heat until steaming but not boiling; stir occasionally.

2. Add the Nutella and whisk until dissolved.

3. Add the Baileys Irish Cream and your chosen CBD option; whisk well to blend.

4. Remove from heat and serve, topped with a dab of the whipped cream.

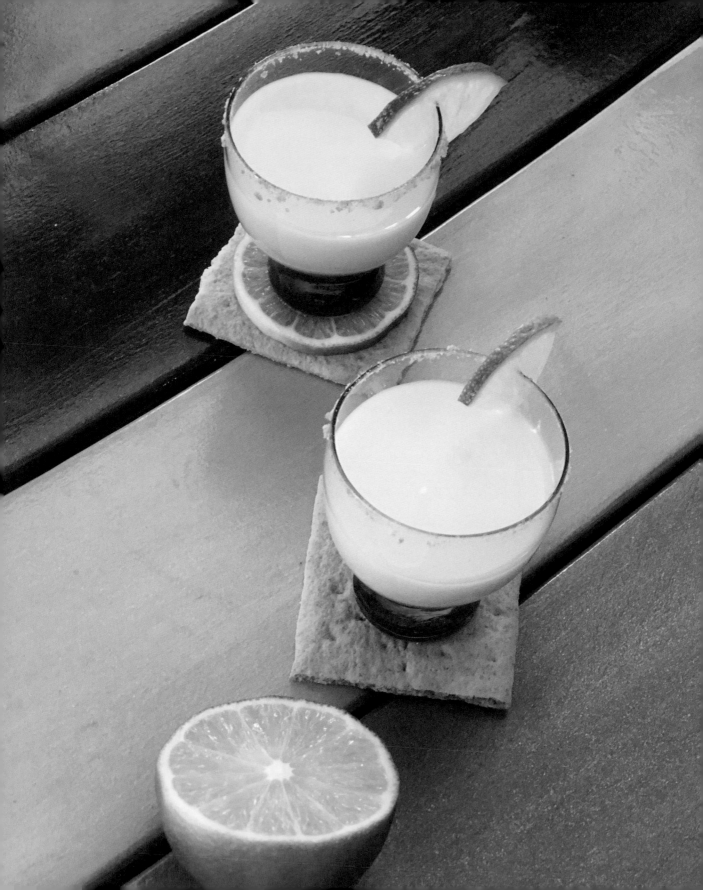

KEY LIME PIE DRINK

This is an easy and deliciously refreshing after-dinner drink. It really does taste like you're drinking key lime pie!

I like to add the water-soluble CBD and the rum or vodka to individual glasses instead of the pitcher. Pour each serving into a metal cocktail shaker; add ice, alcohol, and CBD and mix thoroughly, then pour into a glass. If you have any leftovers, pour them into ice pop trays for a refreshing summer treat. Or make into a slushy by simply combining with ice in a blender until you have the desired consistency. For added nutrition, you can blend in a few tablespoons of hemp seeds.

Total time: 10 minutes | **Makes:** 7 to 10 highball-glass servings

1 (12-ounce) can frozen concentrated limeade

water-soluble CBD (7.5 milliliters for a 60-ounce pitcher)

1 (14-ounce) can sweetened condensed milk (or sweetened hemp milk)

rum (such as Malibu, Bacardi) or vodka of choice

lime slices, whipped cream, or graham crackers, for garnish

1. Add the frozen limeade to a large pitcher, then fill the empty limeade container with water 3 times and add to the pitcher. (This will most likely be less water than the label recommends.)

2. Add the water-soluble CBD and mix well.

3. Add the sweetened condensed milk; stir until well combined.

4. Add alcohol, to taste.

5. Serve over ice with garnishes.

* If you want to make your own limeade, combine 1 cup of fresh lime juice, 1 cup of sugar, and 2 quarts (8 cups) of cold water. Stir well to dissolve the sugar.

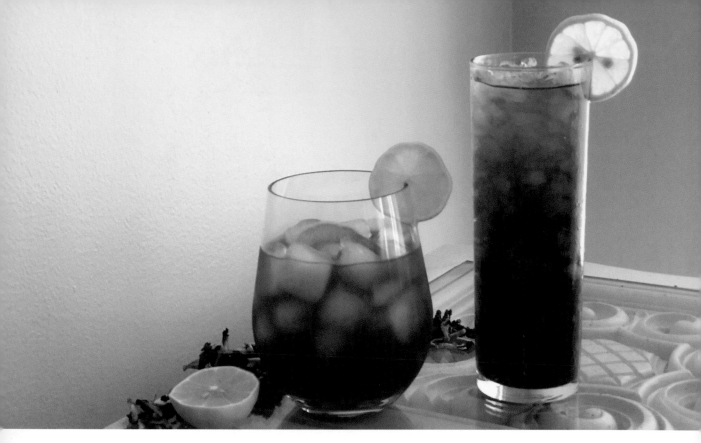

COLOR-CHANGING
CBD SIMPLE SYRUP

This simple syrup will appear navy blue in color because of the butterfly pea flower, best known as the source of blue tea—an herbal tea that changes color depending on the pH level of whatever it's mixed with. When the syrup is mixed with lemon or lemonade, the blue changes to purple. Traditionally mixed with honey, lemon, and ginger, it can be used as a sweetener for Ginger Lemon Tea (page 100) or as a sweetener for alcoholic beverages, and it can also be frozen as ice cubes.

Aside from being a cool party trick, what's nice about the color change is that it instantly tells you when your CBD has been incorporated into your beverage. In addition, the butterfly pea flower contains potent antioxidants.

While butterfly pea flowers might not be found in your grocery store, I found them easily online. Without sugar, the flower tastes like green peas, so you'll definitely want to add sugar unless you want your beverage to taste like green pea soup. If you opt to make this simple syrup with honey, agave, or another sweetener instead of sugar, it will most likely turn purple before it's added to a beverage.

Total time: 10 minutes | **Makes:** 2 cups

COOKING *with* CBD

2 cups boiling water

3 tablespoons dried butterfly pea flowers

½ cup sugar

1 to 2 milliliters water-soluble CBD

1. Boil 2 cups of water. Remove from heat.

2. Let the butterfly blue pea flowers steep in the hot water for 8 minutes.

3. Remove the flower petals with a strainer and then stir in the sugar until it is fully dissolved.

4. Add the CBD and stir well.

5. Place in the refrigerator to cool or in the freezer to solidify. If freezing the CBD simple syrup, pour it into an ice cube tray (preferably silicone) and use as ice cubes. Or pour it into a shallow sheet pan or baking dish, freeze until solid, and scrape with a fork to shave into beverages.

SIMPLE SYRUP WITHOUT THE BUTTERFLY PEA FLOWER

To make traditional simple syrup *without* the butterfly pea flower, simply combine 1 cup of water with 1 cup of sugar in a saucepan and boil until the sugar is dissolved. Remove from the heat and add water-soluble CBD while still warm, stirring well. This is great to use for margaritas, mojitos, lemon drops, and numerous classic cocktails.

You can also use the French press double boiler technique (used to make CBD butter and oil, pages 12–14) to steep hemp flower in sugar water to make simple syrup. Bring 1 cup of water and 1 cup of sugar to boil in the French press; stir to dissolve. Add 1 to 2 grams of CBD flower and simmer over medium low heat for 20 minutes. Reduce the heat again, add ½ to 1 tablespoon of vegetable glycerin for additional sweetening, and simmer for another 5 to 6 minutes. Stir every minute or so to prevent scorching. Remove from heat and strain into a mason jar or other container. Keep refrigerated.

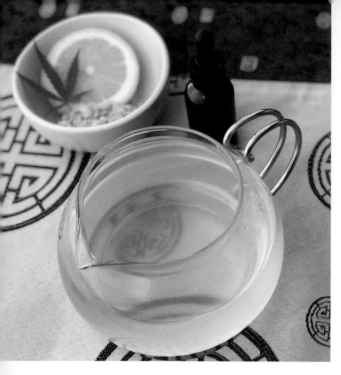

GINGER LEMON TEA

I really enjoy this tea at bedtime. Add some whiskey or bourbon, and you'll have a ginger hot toddy. Or refrigerate it to make a refreshing ginger lemonade.

Prep and cook time: about 25 minutes | **Makes:** 4 servings

2-inch piece ginger root

1 lemon

4 cups water

honey, to taste

2 milliliters water-soluble CBD

1. Wash the ginger root and lemon. Cut the lemon into slices; thinly slice the ginger root.

2. In a small saucepan, bring the water to a boil.

3. Remove from heat and add the ginger and lemon.

4. Steep for 20 minutes, then strain out the lemon and ginger root.

5. Stir in the honey and CBD. Serve warm.

6. For extra CBD and added sweetener, stir in the Color-Changing CBD Simple Syrup (page 98).

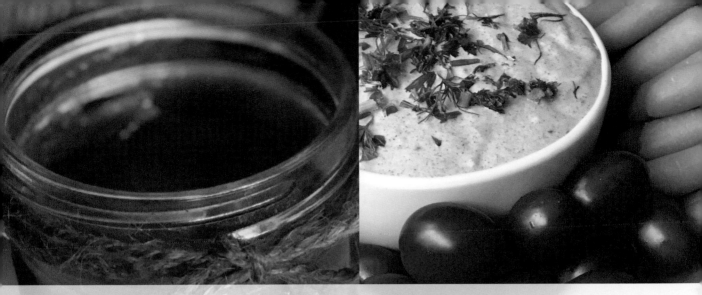

Chapter **7**

DRESSINGS, DIPS, & SAUCES

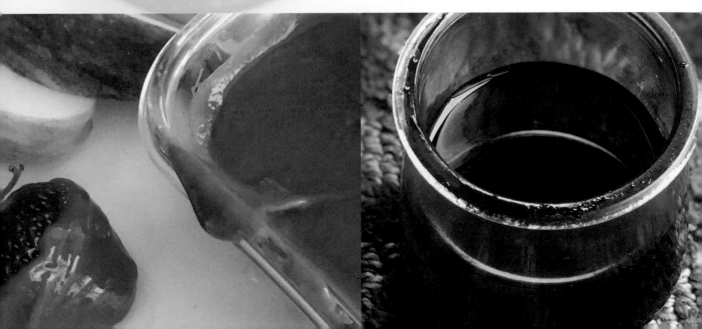

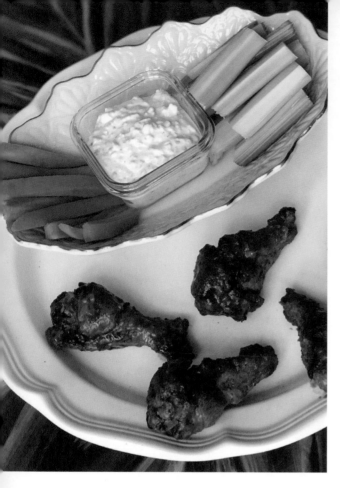

HEMP BLUE CHEESE DRESSING

This is one of those dressings I find a way to use on just about anything, from hot wings to wedge salads to steaks. You can decide to opt out of adding CBD to wings, steak, and so on and use this dressing as your source instead.

Prep and chill time: 15 minutes | **Makes:** 2 to 4 servings

½ cup crumbled blue cheese or Gorgonzola

⅓ cup sour cream

¼ cup mayonnaise

2 cloves garlic, minced

1 tablespoon lemon juice

2 tablespoons hemp seeds

¼ teaspoon pepper

¼ teaspoon salt

CHOOSE ONE OF THE FOLLOWING CBD OPTIONS

- Instead of ¼ cup of mayonnaise, use 2 tablespoons of CBD Homemade Mayonnaise (page 108) + 2 tablespoons of unmedicated mayo; or use ¼ cup of CBD Homemade Mayonnaise.

- Add 1 tablespoon of CBD coconut oil or CBD olive oil.

- Add 1 to 2 milliliters of water-soluble CBD.

1. In a small bowl, combine all the ingredients until well blended.

2. Cover and chill in the refrigerator, or use immediately as a salad dressing, vegetable dip, or dipping sauce for buffalo chicken wings.

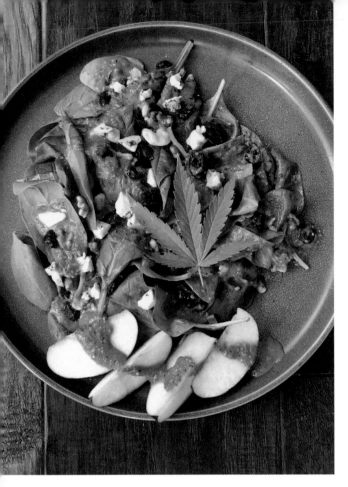

STRAWBERRY HEMP SEED DRESSING

This vinaigrette is sweet and tangy (and gluten free and vegan). The hemp seeds thicken the dressing so that the oil and vinegar won't separate.

I love this dressing on top of a bed of spinach, with blue cheese, walnuts, cranberries, and apple slices. Look for the semi-hard French blue cheese called Fourme d'Ambert. It's one of France's oldest cheeses, dating back to Roman times. Traditionally made from raw cow's milk (but now with pasteurized milk), it has a velvety, almost cream cheese consistency.

Total time: 10 minutes |
Makes: up to 4 servings

1 cup strawberries

2 tablespoons red wine vinegar

1 teaspoon apple cider vinegar

3 tablespoons olive oil

3 tablespoons hemp seeds

CHOOSE ONE OF THE FOLLOWING CBD OPTIONS

• Instead of 3 tablespoons of olive oil, use 1 tablespoon of unmedicated olive oil + 2 tablespoons of CBD olive oil.

• Use 3 tablespoons of CBD olive oil instead of unmedicated olive oil.

• Add 2 milliliters of water-soluble CBD.

1. Combine all the ingredients in a food processor or blender and purée to a smooth consistency.

2. If you don't want to include the CBD in the entire batch, you can make the dressing and then mix water-soluble CBD into an individual serving (.5 milliliter per serving).

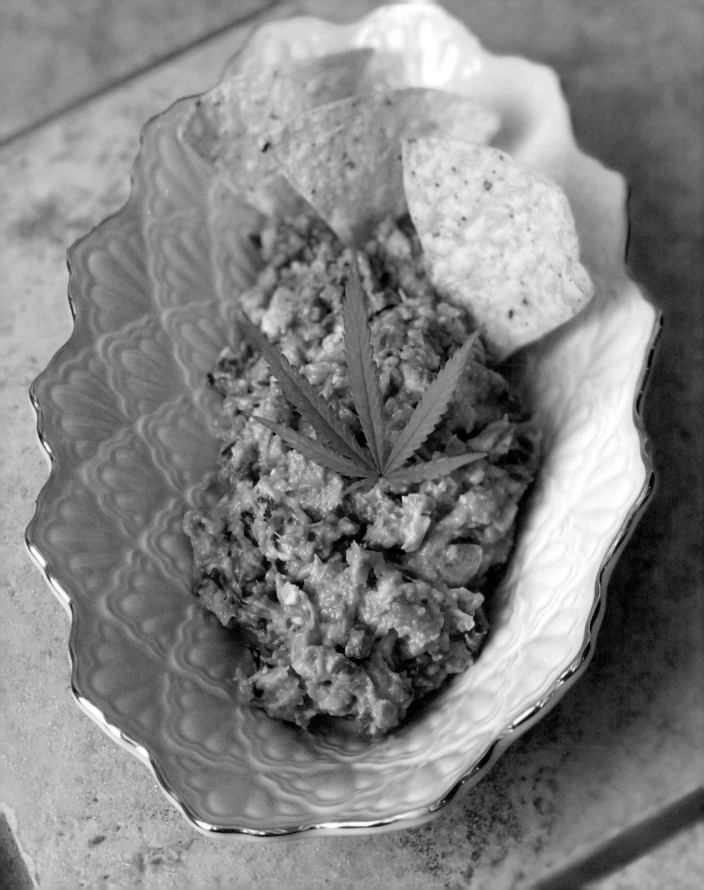

ZESTY GUACAMOLE

Guacamole (or "guac," as it's lovingly referred to in my house), was originally developed by the Aztecs and is a phenomenal source of superfood nutrients. Typically, guac is meant to be served soon after it's made, because avocado turns brown when exposed to air. You can delay this process by pressing plastic wrap over the surface to remove all air bubbles and then storing your guac in the refrigerator. I prefer my guac without garlic, but you can add a minced garlic clove if you wish to ensure that the CBD is fully masked.

Total time: 15 minutes | **Makes:** 2½ cups

juice of 1 or 2 limes

2 large ripe avocados, peeled, pitted, and mashed

1 teaspoon crushed red pepper flakes or ½ jalapeño pepper, seeded and minced

¼ cup minced onion (I prefer white onion)

3 tablespoons chopped fresh cilantro

½ teaspoon salt

CHOOSE ONE OF THE FOLLOWING CBD OPTIONS
- 1 milliliter water-soluble CBD
- 1½ teaspoons CBD hemp seed oil or CBD olive oil

1. Juice a lime and mix half of the juice with the mashed avocado. Add the CBD, mixing until fairly smooth.

2. If using a jalapeño, test its heat by sniffing the minced pieces. Half a pepper should be enough, but if you want it spicier, mince the whole pepper.

3. Add the red pepper flakes or minced jalapeño along with the onion, cilantro, and salt.

4. Taste; if additional lime is needed, add remaining juice from the first lime and mix. Add additional juice from the second lime if preferred.

HOW TO TELL IF YOUR AVOCADO IS RIPE

Ripe avocados are essential for this recipe. Most people gently squeeze the avocado to test for ripeness; if it yields slightly, it's ready to eat. If it feels firm, it needs a day or two, and if it gives too easily, it's overripe. Personally, I prefer the stem method. Pull the stem out of the avocado. If it comes off easily, revealing green or greenish brown underneath, it's ready to eat. If it's hard to remove, the avocado needs a couple more days. If the stem falls off to reveal brown underneath, it's probably overripe—but double-check by using the squeeze method.

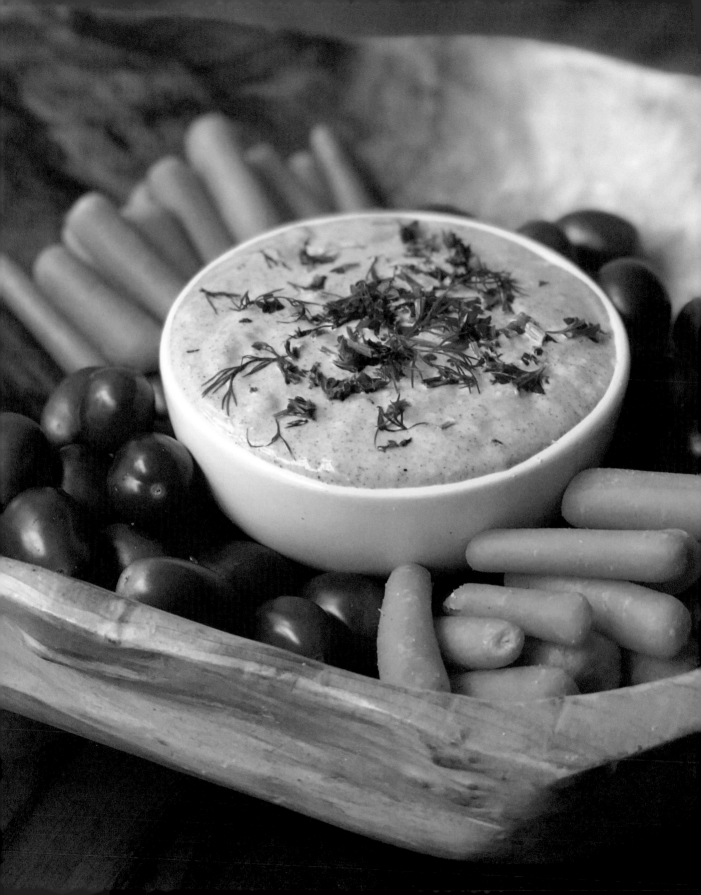

CREAMY HEMP DIPPIN' SAUCE

With the taste and consistency of a creamy Italian dressing, this sauce can be paired with your favorite vegetable platter or a fresh loaf of bread, or you can use it as a dressing for a garden salad. The hemp protein powder gives the sauce a slightly green color. For a non-green hempy dressing, simply make it without the hemp protein powder.

Total time: 10 minutes | **Makes:** 2 servings

½ cup mayonnaise

¼ teaspoon onion powder

2 tablespoons apple cider vinegar

1½ teaspoons sugar

½ teaspoon Italian seasoning

¼ teaspoon garlic powder

¼ teaspoon salt

⅛ teaspoon freshly ground pepper

1 tablespoon hemp seeds

1 tablespoon hemp protein powder

chopped fresh parsley or shredded cheese, as garnish (optional)

CHOOSE ONE OF THE FOLLOWING CBD OPTIONS
- Instead of ½ cup of mayonnaise, use ½ cup of CBD Homemade Mayonnaise (page 108); or use ¼ cup of CBD Homemade Mayonnaise + ¼ cup of unmedicated mayo.
- Add 1 tablespoon of CBD olive oil or CBD hemp seed oil.
- Add 1 to 2.5 milliliters of water-soluble CBD.

1. Combine all of the ingredients except for the garnishes in a blender or food processor. Blend until smooth.

2. Refrigerate, covered, until ready to serve. If you wish, top with chopped parsley or freshly shredded cheese (such as provolone, mozzarella, or Parmesan) for serving.

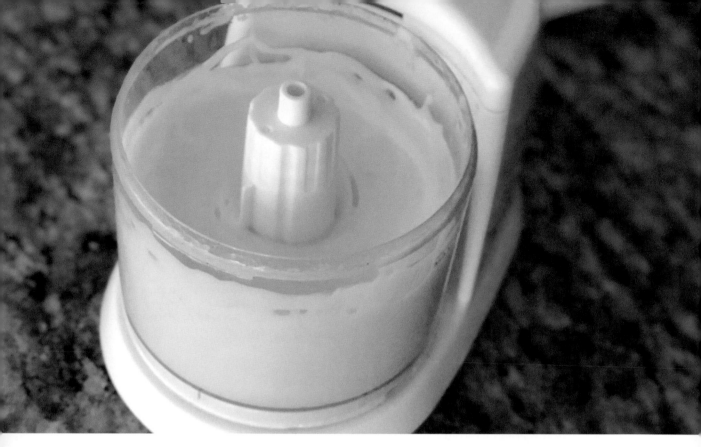

HOMEMADE MAYONNAISE

Once you taste this mayo, you'll wonder why you've never made your own before. It is incredibly easy to make, and it tastes so much better than anything store-bought! Unless you want your mayo to taste like olive oil, go with an extra-light olive oil or a neutral oil without any flavor, such as vegetable oil. I like using apple cider vinegar in this mayonnaise to give it some extra zest and better mask the CBD.

Use the food processor's smaller bowl or the mixture won't have enough contact with the blade and won't emulsify properly. If you don't have a small bowl attachment for your food processor, you can double the recipe to make a larger batch.

Total time: 10 minutes | **Makes:** 1 cup

1 egg, at room temperature

1 tablespoon Dijon mustard or ½ teaspoon dry mustard powder

1 tablespoon red or white wine vinegar or apple cider vinegar, or 2 tablespoons lemon juice (at room temperature)

¼ teaspoon salt, or up to ½ teaspoon if needed

1 cup light cooking oil, such as olive (not extra-virgin), grape seed, safflower, or canola, or more as needed

CHOOSE ONE OF THE FOLLOWING CBD OPTIONS

- Instead of 1 cup of light cooking oil, use ¼ cup of CBD light cooking oil (such as vegetable oil) + ¾ cup of unmedicated light cooking oil.

- Instead of 1 cup of light cooking oil, use 2 tablespoons of CBD light cooking oil + ¾ cup and 2 tablespoons of unmedicated light cooking oil.

- Add 1 to 2.5 milliliters of water-soluble CBD.

1. Add the egg to the small bowl of a food processor and process for 20 seconds.

2. Add the mustard, vinegar or lemon juice, and ¼ teaspoon salt; process for another 20 seconds.

3. Scrape the sides and the bottom of the bowl, if necessary, and slowly drizzle in the oil.

Adding the oil slowly makes for a creamier mayo; total pouring time should be 2 to 3 minutes. When the mixture begins to thicken and emulsify, you can add the remaining oil in a thin stream instead of a drizzle.

4. After all the oil has been added, scrape the bottom and sides of the bowl and process for another 10 seconds.

5. Taste, adding extra salt if needed. If the mayo seems too thin, you can add extra oil to the mixture, based on your preference; turn the processor back on and slowly stream in more oil until it thickens.

6. Transfer the mayo to an airtight container and store in the refrigerator.

QUICK TIP: If for any reason your mayo "breaks" (doesn't mix and starts to curdle), here's how to save it. Just put about a teaspoon of Dijon mustard or an egg yolk in a bowl and slowly beat in the broken mayo until it becomes creamy.

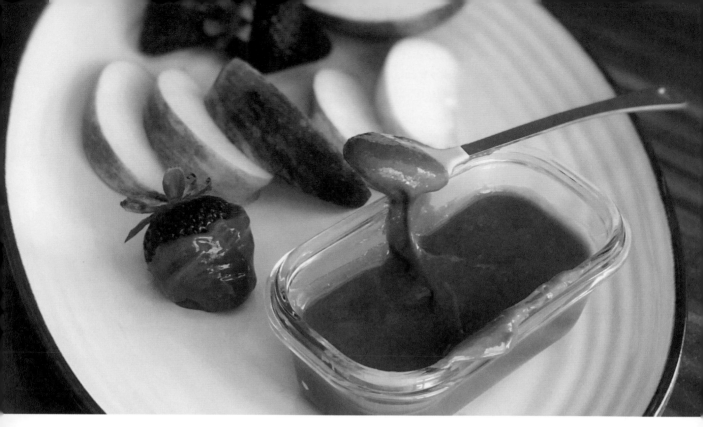

DULCE DE LECHE (DECADENT CARAMEL SAUCE)

This is the easiest way to make your own creamy caramel sauce without creating a gooey mess! It's so easy that I make it at night so that it's ready in the morning for topping pancakes or Make-Ahead French Toast Soufflé (page 20).

I recommend going light on the CBD that you add to this sauce, as the flavor isn't strong enough on its own to mask a large amount. You can make it *without* CBD and then add it to your serving when you mix your Dulce de Leche into a morning coffee, breakfast dish, or dessert. The sauce will thicken slightly once you add the CBD and refrigerate it.

Prep and bake time: 1 hour and 35 minutes | **Makes:** 1¼ cups

1 (14- to 15-ounce) can sweetened condensed milk

CHOOSE ONE OF THE FOLLOWING CBD OPTIONS
- **1 milliliter water-soluble CBD (recommended)**
- **1½ teaspoons CBD vegetable oil**

1. Preheat the oven to 425°F, with a rack in the middle position. While the oven heats, pour the sweetened condensed milk into an 8x8-inch oven-safe dish (can be a small pie plate). Cover tightly with foil.

2. Set the dish containing the condensed milk in a roasting pan or other oven-safe pan (about 9x13-inch). Add enough hot water to the outer pan to reach halfway to three-quarters up the sides of the foil-covered dish.

3. Place on the middle rack of the oven and bake for 45 minutes. Then check the water level in the outer pan and add more water if needed.

4. Bake for 45 minutes longer, then turn off the heat but leave the milk in the hot oven. (You can leave it there for another hour.)

5. When cool enough to handle easily, remove the pans from the oven and add CBD to the warm milk (now a dark caramel color). Pour the milk into a bowl and use an emulsion blender (recommended) or electric mixer to get rid of any small lumps that may have formed while the milk was cooking.

6. Store in an airtight container in the refrigerator for up to 1 month. Texture will be thick like pudding and may congeal to a slightly thicker consistency after adding the CBD and refrigerating. Can eat it cold or reheat.

WHAT'S THE DIFFERENCE?

You may wonder how a dulce de leche sauce is different from caramel sauce. Dulce de leche is typically made with condensed milk and simmered for hours, while caramel sauce is a reduced mixture of water, sugar, heavy whipping cream, and butter. Dulce de leche originated in Latin America—the name is Spanish for "candy [made] of milk," or "caramel." Both are used in the same way but the process of making them is different (the consistency, color, and taste can vary.)

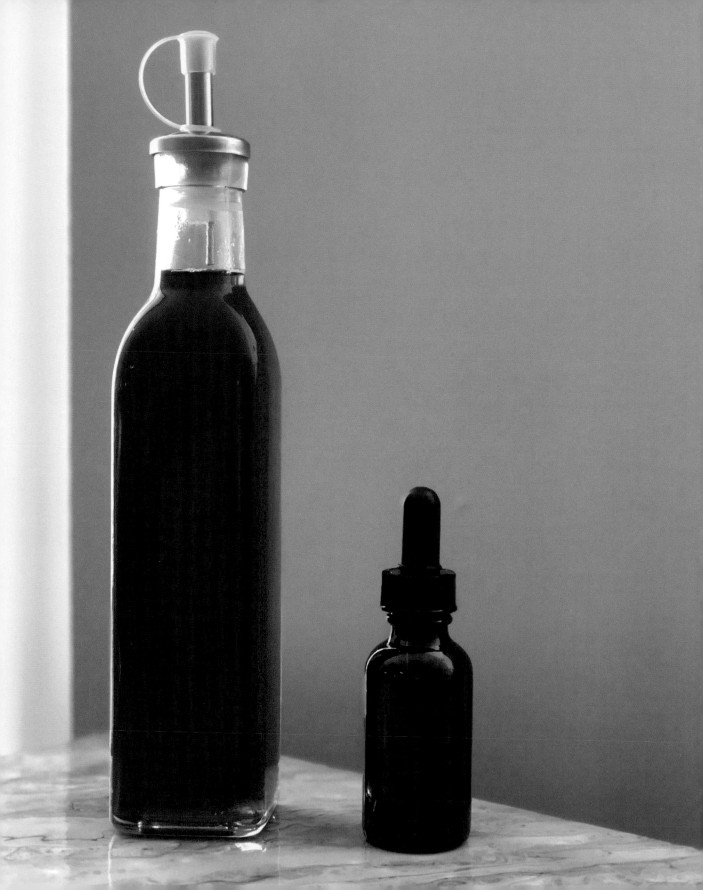

STRAWBERRY SYRUP

Water-soluble CBD works best for this syrup, since there's no fat substance such as milk or butter into which CBD oil can be mixed. However, you can use decarbed CBD flower to make CBD Strawberry Syrup (or maple syrup or honey) in a French press—see the sidebar for instructions.

Prep and cook time: 25 minutes | **Makes:** 2 to 4 servings

1 cup chopped strawberries

½ cup water

¼ cup sugar

.5 to 1 milliliter water-soluble CBD

1. Put the chopped strawberries in a small saucepan and add the water.

2. Over medium heat, bring to a simmer and cook until the water is bright pink and the strawberries are mushy, about 10 minutes.

3. Strain out the strawberries and return the pink water to the stovetop.

4. Add the sugar, bring to a simmer over medium heat, and continue cooking until the syrup begins to thicken, about 5 to 10 minutes.

5. Since the syrup will thicken more as it cools, test it by taking a small amount on a spoon and blowing on it to cool it. When you're happy with the consistency, remove the syrup from the heat, stir in the CBD, and set aside to cool.

6. Transfer the cooled syrup to an airtight container and refrigerate or serve right away on pancakes or waffles.

CBD SYRUP IN A FRENCH PRESS

Here's how to use a French press to infuse syrup or honey with CBD. Combine 3.5 grams of decarbed CBD flower with 1 cup of syrup or honey inside the French press, but don't press down on the plunger. Set the French press in a pot of boiling water on the stovetop. Use a candy thermometer to ensure that the syrup stays at around 160°F, so that it simmers but never comes to a full boil. Add water to the outer pot if necessary to reduce the heat or reduce the heat slightly if the water continues to boil.

Let the hemp flower steep in the hot syrup for at least 40 minutes, lifting the French press from the water occasionally to stir the mixture. After 40 minutes to an hour, remove the French press from the water and press down on the plunger. Pour the syrup into a glass jar and let it cool to room temperature. Serve or refrigerate.

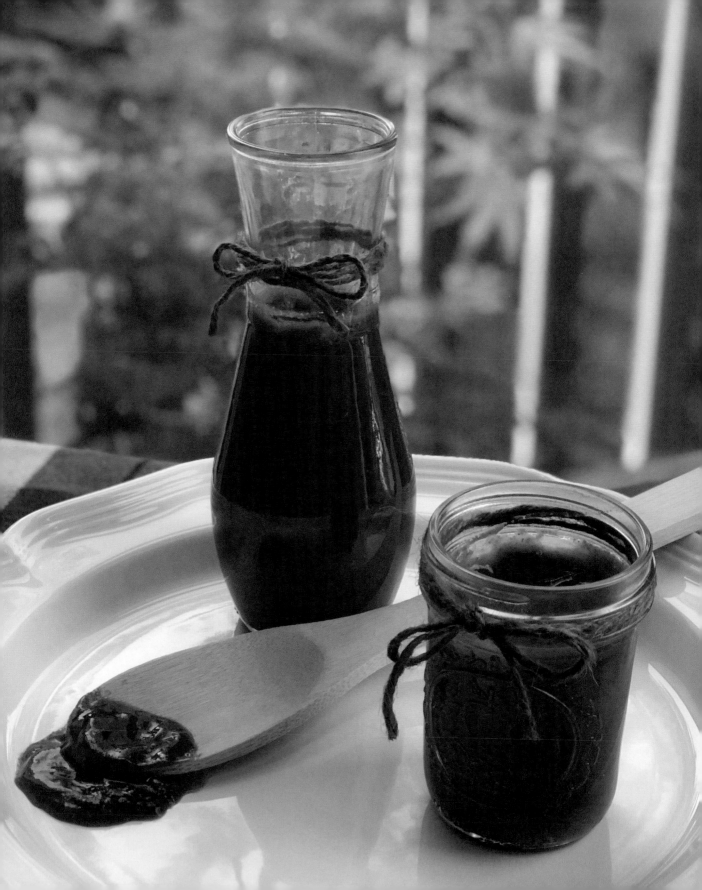

SAINT LOUIS–STYLE BBQ SAUCE

My husband was born and raised in St. Louis. When we were dating, he made this BBQ sauce for his fall-off-the-bone pork ribs. It's perfect for smothering onto just about anything—from chicken to pork to steak to meatloaf (see page 67). Because the sauce contains sugar, it can burn at high temperatures and should only be used when the meat is over low heat, or at the end of its cooking time. Since CBD can't handle high heat, either, the sauce is perfect for infusing with CBD.

For most of the recipes in this book, you can substitute ingredients and still get great results. That's not the case with this sauce. When I've subbed something out, gone without an ingredient, or changed it slightly (like adding minced garlic instead of garlic powder), I've always regretted it.

Total time: 1 hour | **Makes:** 3½ cups

2 cups ketchup

½ cup water

⅓ cup apple cider vinegar

⅓ cup brown sugar

2 tablespoons yellow mustard

1 tablespoon onion powder

1 tablespoon garlic powder

1 tablespoon Worcestershire sauce

½ teaspoon cayenne pepper

¼ teaspoon salt

CHOOSE ONE OF THE FOLLOWING CBD OPTIONS
- 2 to 3 milliliters water-soluble CBD (recommended)
- 2 tablespoons CBD olive, vegetable, or coconut oil
- 1 tablespoon CBD butter

1. In a medium saucepan over low heat, combine all the ingredients except the CBD. Let simmer, stirring occasionally, for 20 minutes. The sauce should be thin but not watery.

2. Stir in the CBD. Remove from heat and let cool for 20 to 30 minutes.

3. The sauce is ready as soon as it has cooled, but it tastes better after it is refrigerated and even better if it sits for a day in the refrigerator.

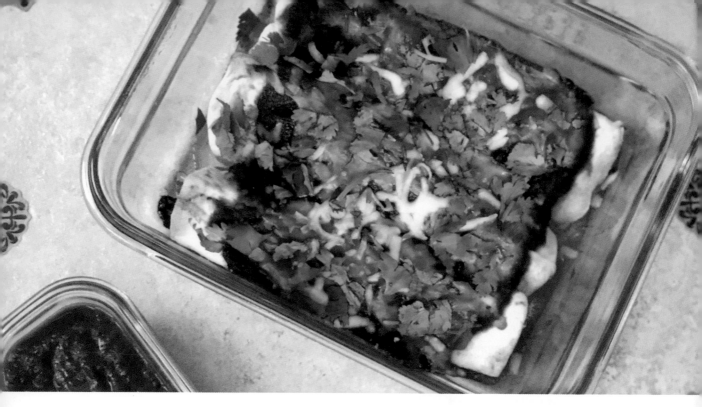

EVERYDAY ENCHILADA SAUCE

Be sure to taste your chili powder before incorporating it into this enchilada sauce, since it will definitely influence the overall flavor of the sauce. If your sauce ends up being too spicy for your taste, reduce the heat to low and whisk in 1 to 2 tablespoons of butter. You can also add CBD butter this way, if more CBD is needed.

Perfect for making chicken enchiladas, this sauce is also delicious on eggs (huevos rancheros, anyone?). As a quick breakfast, take sauce left over from dinner and smother it onto Egg-in-the-Basket Avocado Toast (page 25).

Prep and cook time: 15 minutes | **Makes:** 1½ cups

2 tablespoons vegetable oil

1 tablespoon onion powder

1 tablespoon minced garlic

¼ cup finely chopped red bell pepper

2 teaspoons chili powder

1 teaspoon ground cumin

¼ teaspoon cayenne pepper

1 beef bouillon cube (not combined with water)

½ cup chicken or vegetable broth

2 (8-ounce) cans tomato sauce

¼ teaspoon salt

¼ teaspoon black pepper

COOKING *with* CBD

CHOOSE ONE OF THE FOLLOWING CBD OPTIONS
- Add 2 milliliters of water-soluble CBD.
- Add 1 tablespoon of CBD vegetable oil.

1. Heat the vegetable oil in a nonstick medium saucepan over medium heat. Add the onion powder, garlic, and bell pepper and cook until the vegetables are soft, about 1 to 2 minutes.

2. Add the chili powder, cumin, cayenne, and bouillon cube along with the chicken or vegetable broth.

3. Cook, stirring, until the liquid thickens slightly, about 2 minutes.

4. Add the tomato sauce, salt, and pepper, and stir until well combined; cook for 5 more minutes.

5. Reduce heat to low and add the CBD.

6. Purée with an immersion blender on low speed until smooth or remove from heat and transfer to a blender to purée.

MOJO CHICKEN ENCHILADAS

Combine this enchilada sauce with tortillas and Mojo Shredded Slow Cooker Chicken (page 65), and dinner is made! Use tongs to lift the cooked chicken onto flour tortillas, then roll each tortilla around the filling and place seam-side down in an 8x8-inch or larger baking dish. (An 8x8-inch pan will hold 4 enchiladas.)

Top the tortillas with enchilada sauce until well coated, then add shredded cheese, such as queso or cotija. Heat in a 250°F oven for 10 minutes or less until the cheese is melted and the tortillas are slightly crispy on the edges. Serve with extra cheese and your toppings of choice, such as sour cream and chopped cilantro.

CONVERSION CHARTS

VOLUME

U.S.	U.S. Equivalent	Metric
1 tablespoon (3 teaspoons)	½ fluid ounce	15 milliliters
¼ cup	2 fluid ounces	60 milliliters
⅓ cup	3 fluid ounces	90 milliliters
½ cup	4 fluid ounces	120 milliliters
⅔ cup	5 fluid ounces	150 milliliters
¾ cup	6 fluid ounces	180 milliliters
1 cup	8 fluid ounces	240 milliliters
2 cups	16 fluid ounces	480 milliliters

WEIGHT

U.S.	Metric
½ ounce	15 grams
1 ounce	30 grams
2 ounces	60 grams
¼ pound	115 grams
⅓ pound	150 grams
½ pound	225 grams
¾ pound	350 grams
1 pound	450 grams

TEMPERATURE

Fahrenheit (°F)	Celsius (°C)	Fahrenheit (°F)	Celsius (°C)
70°F	20°C	220°F	105°C
100°F	40°C	240°F	115°C
120°F	50°C	260°F	125°C
130°F	55°C	280°F	140°C
140°F	60°C	300°F	150°C
150°F	65°C	325°F	165°C
160°F	70°C	350°F	175°C
170°F	75°C	375°F	190°C
180°F	80°C	400°F	200°C
190°F	90°C	425°F	220°C
200°F	95°C	450°F	230°C

CBD 101: YOUR CANNABIDIOL REFERENCE GUIDE

WHAT IS CANNABIDIOL?

Cannabidiol—CBD—is one of at least 113 cannabinoid compounds found in the buds (or flowers) of cannabis plants. While both hemp and marijuana contain CBD, the cannabinoid is most abundant in hemp. CBD is known as a non-psychoactive compound, which means it doesn't produce the "high" associated with THC, but it does carry some of the same medicinal benefits. There are other non-psychoactive cannabinoids such as CBG (cannabigerol), CBC (cannabichromene), and CBDV (cannabidivarin) that host a variety of positive health effects similar to CBD, but they're not as well known or as widely used as CBD at this time.

Anthropologists have chronicled over 6,000 years of documented uses for cannabis—from food to textiles to medicinal applications, with China's *Pen-ts'ao ching*, the world's oldest medical book, or pharmacopoeia, as the first to mention cannabis. The origin of the Pen-ts'ao has been traced back to Emperor Shen-nung's dynasty, 2700 BC. This pharmacopoeia is the oldest collection of instructions for compounding specific drugs, plus their uses and effects. Among them are over 100 medical uses for cannabis, including memory problems, malaria, rheumatism, and gout.[5] While this is centuries before scientists discovered specific compounds in cannabis and how they worked, ancient texts from the Chinese, the Assyrians, and the Hindu religion all recognized the plant's therapeutic uses.

WHY DOES CBD HELP SO MANY CONDITIONS?

Much of what we know today about CBD stems from the research of Israeli chemist Raphael Mechoulam, whose breakthrough discoveries from the early 1960s were the first steps in understanding the effects of individual cannabinoids, including CBD and THC. Mechoulam continues researching cannabis today, and now there is a vast collection of scientific papers, medical reports, and anecdotal evidence indicating that CBD can help more than 50 health conditions, including the following:

---

5 Andrew Hand et al., "History of Medical Cannabis," *Journal of Pain and Symptom Management* 9, no. 4 (2016): 387–94, https://medreleaf.com/app/uploads/2018/03/1.History-of-medical-cannabis.pdf?fbclid=IwAR0k6mOT9ZiR4Kc2isz HmmbyHpkZvEBvpM7_DMAmnU0TZ8zMPbtztT41WBU.

Acne

ADD/ADHD

Addiction

ALS

Alzheimer's disease

Anorexia

Anxiety

Atherosclerosis

Arthritis

Asthma

Autism

Bipolar affective disorder

Cancer

Crohn's disease and colitis

Depression

Endocrine disorders

Epilepsy and seizures

Fibromyalgia

Glaucoma

Heart disease

Huntington's disease

Inflammation

Irritable bowel syndrome

Kidney disease

Liver disease

Lyme disease

Menstrual cramps

Metabolic syndrome

Migraines

Mood disorder

Motion sickness

Multiple sclerosis

Nausea

Neurodegeneration

Neuropathic pain

Obesity

OCD

Parkinson's disease

Prion-MCD

PTSD

Rheumatism

Schizophrenia

Sickle cell anemia

Skin conditions

Sleep disorders

Spinal cord injury

Stress

Stroke/TBI

Thyroid disease

CBD has so many benefits because it stimulates the endocannabinoid system, or ECS, a cell-signaling bodily system identified by Dr. Mechoulam in the 1990s. Scientists are still studying the ECS, but the primary role is to promote homeostasis among all bodily functions. The ECS processes our sense of appetite, our sense of pain, even our moods; it processes our basic brain functions, balance, movement, learning and memory, motor control, sleep, stress, digestion, metabolism, inflammation, and other immune system responses. It also mediates the effects of cannabis.

When CBD enters the body, it helps the endocannabinoid system balance deficiencies and adjust excessive activity. Essentially, CBD nudges the ECS to work harder to bring homeostasis to the body. Depending on what's out of whack, that translates to CBD assisting in relieving depression, lowering inflammation, lowering blood pressure, improving sleep, or reducing anxiety and pain.

IS CBD LEGAL?

If the CBD comes from the hemp plant, then yes, it's federally legal. The 2018 U.S. Farm Bill legalized hemp as an agricultural commodity. The legislation defined hemp plants and hemp products that contain .3% THC or less federally legal.

If the CBD comes from marijuana, then it's only legal in states that have legalized marijuana. Marijuana is defined as containing much more than .3% THC, and that's still federally illegal.

While the legalization of hemp-derived CBD is relatively new, doctors in the United States did prescribed cannabis medication in liquid form (until the passing of the 1937 Marijuana Tax Act); the liquid cannabis was used primarily for pain management but also for a variety of other ailments including whooping cough. In 2018 the FDA approved the first prescription drug containing CBD, called Epidiolex, used to treat two epilepsy disorders—Lennox-Gastaut syndrome and Dravet syndrome. For patients at least two years old, the drug is taken orally with food (usually twice a day) as prescribed by a doctor.

HEMP-DERIVED CBD OIL

The CBD extraction process includes high-tech CO_2 or ethanol extraction equipment designed to isolate the cannabinoids in the raw hemp flower and turn them into oil. Extracted CBD oil is typically sold in a small bottle with a dropper that indicates dosages in milliliters. It can also be infused into various products, from skin lotions to bath bombs to food.

- Full-spectrum CBD refers to the full plant extract. This means all of the cannabinoids in the hemp flower were extracted, including terpenes, THC, and other compounds that occur naturally in the cannabis plant. That small amount of THC (.3% or less) carries medicinal benefits but won't cause psychoactive effects. Full-spectrum CBD is also sold in concentrated forms such as shatter, dabs, and resin, which are typically vaped or used in products such as lotions and bath bombs.

- Broad-spectrum CBD is full-spectrum CBD that has undergone an additional extraction process to remove all trace amounts of THC. It still contains the complete profile of cannabinoids, terpenes, and other natural compounds, but no THC.

- CBD isolate contains pure CBD only; it does not contain any other cannabinoids, terpenes, or other natural compounds found in hemp. Usually CBD isolate is purchased as a white powder (what it looks like when it's extracted), or it may be hardened into a slab, rock, or crystal. Since it's tasteless and odorless, CBD isolate can be used to create a variety of products.

QUICK TIP: Water-soluble CBD is another option available in full spectrum, broad spectrum, and CBD isolate. It can be purchased in powder form or in a liquid (but is typically purchased as a liquid).

You can also legally purchase CBD hemp flower (the bud of the hemp plant) to smoke or to infuse into cooking oil or butter (more on that in Chapter 1).

WHICH KIND OF CBD SHOULD I USE?

There isn't an easy answer as to which type of CBD will work best for a particular person, because it depends on various factors including the severity and type of condition it's being used to treat (chronic pain, anxiety, seizures, acne, etc.). For pain and inflammation, many CBD patients find a dual approach most effective. CBD lotion, salve, or topical oil is applied to the skin to give immediate relief, and the patient also ingests CBD oil to address the inflammation from the inside.

Researchers initially assumed that CBD in its isolated form is more potent and concentrated than full-spectrum CBD. However, the opposite is actually true. CBD isolate doesn't work as efficiently as full-spectrum CBD when administered at the same dose. While both forms do work, full-spectrum CBD produces better anti-inflammatory results for a longer period of time and at a lower dosage.[6] This is due to what is called the "entourage effect"—a phrase coined by researchers to describe the way cannabis compounds work together in the human body. Basically, CBD by itself isn't as effective as when all the cannabinoids (such as CBG and CBC) are able to work together. As the saying goes, *for CBD to be the most effective, it needs an entourage!*

So while CBD isolate and full-spectrum CBD produce similar results, the synergistic effects of CBD paired with all phytocompounds in the hemp plant is what's most effective. Even for treatment-resistant epilepsy, the entourage effect of full-spectrum CBD works better than CBD isolate, which is why the medication Epidiolex isn't comprised solely of CBD.[7]

Here's what to consider when choosing what kind of CBD to use:

- Full-spectrum CBD offers the full entourage effect, with .3% THC or less. This is the most natural form of CBD oil with the least amount of manufacturing, which is why it has a strong (bitter) odor and taste.

- Broad-spectrum CBD contains no THC but offers an entourage effect from all the other cannabinoids it contains.

- CBD isolate is pure CBD without any other cannabinoids. Since it doesn't contain THC or any other cannabinoids, it doesn't deliver the entourage effect.

---

6 Ruth Gallily, Zhannah Yekhtin, and Lumír Ondřej Hanuš, "Overcoming the Bell-Shaped Dose-Response of Cannabidiol by Using Cannabis Extract Enriched in Cannabidiol," *Scientific Research* 6, no. 2 (February 2015): 75–85, https://m.scirp.org/papers/53912.

7 Fabrício A. Pamplona, Lorenzo Rolim da Silva, and Ana Carolina Coan, "Corrigendum: Potential Clinical Benefits of CBD-Rich Cannabis Extracts Over Purified CBD in Treatment-Resistant Epilepsy: Observational Data Meta-Analysis," *Frontiers in Neurology* 9 (January 2019), https://www.researchgate.net/publication/330288128_Corrigendum_Potential_Clinical_Benefits_of_CBD-Rich_Cannabis_Extracts_Over_Purified_CBD_in_Treatment-Resistant_Epilepsy_Observational_Data_Meta-analysis.

HOW MUCH SHOULD I TAKE?

Some people take CBD in the morning to relieve pain, some people take it at night to help them sleep, and some people take it throughout the day. A recommended daily dosage will be listed on the CBD oil bottle. For instance, a full-spectrum water-soluble CBD dose is typically .5 milliliter twice a day, which can equate to 10 milligrams of CBD for the entire day. Manufacturers suggest that if there isn't a noticeable change in your condition, you can scale up by increments of .25 or .5 milliliter. If you feel overly tired (typically the main side effect from taking too much), you can scale back.

CBD DOSAGE CALCULATORS

Free calculators are available online to give a ballpark figure for overall CBD dosage based on ailments and body weight. One of these is found at https://cbddosagecalculator.com (calculations are based on research studies). Apps such as Hemp Dispensing Calculator and Releaf are also great tools.

Though CBD calculators base the dosage on the severity of ailments and on body weight, sometimes body weight isn't a direct correlation to proper dosage. Everyone is different, plus store-bought brands of CBD vary in concentration, so it may take some time to find the right amount for you. If you find the recommended dose ineffective, you can scale up; if you're seeing results but aren't sure if you're taking too much, you can try dialing it back to see if it still works.

Math is not my strong point, and sometimes I find myself having difficulties calculating the correct CBD dosage in a recipe or serving size. Luckily, there are online calculators that will do the work for you. Here are two of them:

https://wakeandbake.co/thc-dosage-calculator

https://jeffthe420chefcalculator.com

CALCULATING CBD POTENCY IN OIL AND BUTTER

Follow these steps to determine the amount of CBD in your butter or oil, and how much is in a serving of food:

1. Start with the CBD percentage in your hemp flower: _____ %

2. Divide that percentage by 100 to get the total CBD per gram:

_____ % ÷ 100 = _____ CBD/gram

3. Multiply the CBD/gram by 1,000 to get the number of milligrams of CBD per gram:

_____ CBD/gram x 1,000 = _____milligrams CBD/gram

4. Now multiply that number by the total weight of the CBD flower used:

_____milligrams CBD/gram x _____ grams cannabis = _____ total milligrams CBD

5. Divide that batch number by the amount of oil or butter (in milliliters):

_____ milligrams CBD ÷ _____ milliliters butter = _____ milligrams CBD/milliliters butter

6. To calculate how much CBD will be in a recipe, take the amount of butter or cooking oil you infused...

_____ milliliters butter in recipe x _____ milligrams CBD/milliliters butter = _____ milligrams CBD in recipe

... and divide that by the number of servings you're making:

_____ milligrams CBD in recipe ÷ _____ servings = _____ milligrams CBD per serving

As an example, let's infuse 3.5 grams of a 15% CBD strain into 1 cup (250 milliliters) butter. Here are the answers to the above steps:

1. 15% CBD

2. 15% CBD ÷ 100 = 0.15 CBD/gram

3. 0.15 CBD/gram x 1,000 = 150 milligrams CBD

4. 150 milligram CBD x 3.5 grams in the batch = 525 milligrams total CBD (the amount of CBD infused into the butter or oil)

5. 525 milligrams CBD ÷ 250 milliliters (1 cup) butter = 2.1 CBD milligrams per milliliter butter

Taking that a step further, there are 16 tablespoons in 1 cup of butter. To find out how much CBD is in 1 tablespoon:

- 1 cup butter = 16 tablespoons
- 1 tablespoon butter = 14.79 milliliters
- 2.1 CBD/milligrams x 14.79 milliliters = 31.059 milligrams CBD per 1 tablespoon butter

If you know there are approximately 31 milligrams CBD in each tablespoon, you'll be able to figure out how many tablespoons of CBD butter to add versus how much unmedicated butter to add if a recipe calls for both.

6. To calculate Step 6, let's say we're using this batch of CBD butter to make cookies. Here's how to calculate how much CBD is in each cookie if the recipe yields 25 cookies and calls for 1 cup butter. Your 1 cup CBD butter contains 525 milligrams CBD, so you know that you'll be baking with 525 milligrams CBD.

- 250 milliliters butter (1 cup) x 2.1 CBD milligrams/milliliters = 525 milligrams CBD
- 525 milligrams CBD ÷ 25 cookies = 2 milligrams CBD per cookie

You can also use one of the dosage calculators available online (see page 123).

CAN I OVERDOSE?

There really isn't any research indicating that it's possible to overdose from CBD or that CBD has extremely negative side effects, particularly because it is non-psychoactive and nonaddictive. But studies do show that you can hit a plateau with CBD isolate, meaning that if you take too much at a time, the increased dose won't do anything additional and may actually cause the CBD to stop working. This means that you can dose yourself out of CBD isolate's effectiveness by taking too much at once.[8]

On the other hand, CBD rich-extract (full-spectrum CBD or broad-spectrum CBD) *won't* lose effectiveness as the dose is increased. You might feel dizzy, lightheaded, or sleepy from taking too much, but the medication will continue to work until it naturally wears off as it leaves your system. There's also indications that long-term use of CBD can actually result in reverse tolerance depending on the condition. Tolerance occurs when a person no longer responds to a drug and needs to take a higher dose to achieve the same level of effectiveness, but this isn't necessarily the case with CBD. For example, there's a substantial amount of scientific research supporting the use of CBD as a treatment for inflammation and inflammatory pain. If you're taking CBD regularly to reduce inflammation and it's working, then that means the inflammation is decreasing, so with less inflammation, a lesser amount of CBD is needed to combat it.[9]

ARE THERE ANY SIDE EFFECTS?

In 2017 the European Industrial Hemp Association commissioned a review of side effects from 132 scientific studies examining CBD as a treatment for epilepsy and other conditions, including Alzheimer's disease and drug dependency. The review, titled *An Update on Safety and Side Effects of Cannabidiol:*

---

8   Ruth Gallily et al., "Overcoming the Bell-Shaped Dose-Response of Cannabidiol."
9   J. D. Nguyen et al., "Tolerance to Hypothermic and Atinoceptive Effects of THC Vapor Inhalation in Rats," *Pharmacology Biochemistry and Behavior* 172 (September 2018): 33–38, https://www.ncbi.nlm.nih.gov/pubmed/30031028.

A Review of Clinical Data and Relevant Animal Studies, was to determine the most commonly reported side effects experienced by the participants in these studies (including mice and humans).

Overall, the review determined that as CBD was administered at higher and higher dosages, human participants experienced the following side effects: tiredness, diarrhea, and changes in appetite/weight. Some participants found that using CBD with other medications made those medications more effective; others found CBD made the medications less effective. However, the subjects in these studies were all given greater quantities of CBD than what the average person would consume. In some of the studies, participants took 300 milligrams of CBD on the first day and then 600 milligrams of CBD the next day; others took 600 milligrams every day for 30 days; some took 300 milligrams for 6 weeks.

In a double-blind, placebo-controlled study published in 2018 and funded by GW Research Ltd., CBD was administered to participants in three different ways:

1. Single ascending dose (at 1,500, 3,000, 4,500, or 6,000 milligrams CBD)

2. Multiple dose (750 or 1,500 milligrams twice daily)

3. In food (1,500 milligrams CBD single dose).

The most common adverse effects identified in this study were diarrhea, nausea, headache, and somnolence, but researchers concluded that oral administration of CBD at doses up to 6,000 milligrams "was well tolerated" by all participants. Interestingly, the study concluded that *food* offers the best delivery system for CBD: "Food increased the bioavailability of CBD and, as such, administering CBD with food would maximize bioavailability and likely reduce within-day fluctuation [of CBD]."[10]

So to get the most out of your CBD, put it in your food. And if you want consistent results, *keep* putting it in your food.

DOES THE ORIGIN OR BRAND OF CBD MATTER?

As a substance, CBD is extremely safe—but not all CBD is the same quality, depending on where it comes from and how it was manufactured.

HEMP-DERIVED CBD. When you purchase hemp-derived CBD, ask for batch-testing lab reports to show that it is void of contaminants. Hemp for food or for CBD can legally be grown only on agricultural

---

10 Lesley Taylor et al., "A Phase I, Randomized, Double-Blind, Placebo-Controlled, Single Ascending Dose, Multiple Dose, and Food Effect Trial of the Safety, Tolerability, and Pharmacokinetics of Highly Purified Cannabidiol in Healthy Subjects," *CNS Drugs* 32, no. 11 (October 2018): 1053–67, https://www.ncbi.nlm.nih.gov/pmc/articles/PMC6223703.

land, so lab reports will show that the CBD is safe to consume. The lab report will also tell you the percentages of cannabinoids, so you'll be able to verify the amount of THC and CBD.

In 2019, the hemp industry also introduced an initiative to provide high standards, best practices, and self-regulation known as the US Hemp Authority Certification Program. A list of companies that have met these standards can be found online at https://www.ushempauthority.org/certified-companies.

CBD DERIVED FROM MARIJUANA. If marijuana is legal in your state, all products sold in dispensaries go through a state or local approval process to check for pesticides and other contaminants. Lab results will indicate that the marijuana is essentially grown organically (without the use of chemical pesticides).

You can also ask if a dispensary is vertically integrated, or "seed-to-consumer," which means the business oversees every aspect of the marijuana it sells and therefore has greater quality control. Vertically integrated cannabis companies know exactly where the seed came from, how it was grown, and how it was processed or extracted. There are also CBD-hemp companies that are virtually integrated.

INGREDIENTS AFFECTING POTENCY. The final point to consider is the amount of CBD in the product you are purchasing. CBD is marketed as all-natural with no added ingredients, but if you're buying CBD with added flavors to mask the bitterness, you should ask what kind of preservatives are being used, and how much. Some manufacturers use vegetable glycerin or other oils to thin and dilute CBD oil for vaping. Some people may be allergic to these additives—and, of course, adding them means less CBD in the bottle.

ACKNOWLEDGMENTS

Many thanks to my husband Andrew, who kept the house well stocked with hemp flower and valuable words of advice throughout this process.

Thank you to my daughter for being so patient with me as I turned our kitchen into the battleground for many successful and failed experiments, and for accepting the fact that in our house it's absolutely normal for Mom to take many, many, many photos of food.

To the talented Rocio Martinez of Rocio Beauty Pixels, thank you for taking such beautiful photos of my daughter (and me) for this book. (And to Tami for recommending Rocio!)

To all my friends and family—thank you for being my taste testers and giving me your honest feedback and support.

Special thanks to Matt and Mike of American Shaman of Oakville for introducing me to CBD Water Soluble and to Olivia and the makers of LEVO, who sent me the LEVO II to test out for this book.

Thank you to Ulysses Press for granting me the opportunity to write *Cooking with CBD*.

ABOUT THE AUTHOR

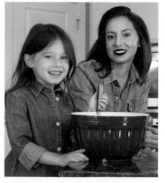

JEN HOBBS is a graduate of Fairleigh Dickinson University's MFA program. She's the author of *American Hemp: How Growing Our Newest Cash Crop Can Improve Our Health, Clean Our Environment, and Slow Climate Change* and the coauthor of *Jesse Ventura's Marijuana Manifesto*. This is her first cookbook, but the kitchen isn't the only place she's dabbled in cannabis-infused edibles. She's also experienced some of the most popular munchies in cannabis culture, ranging from Amsterdam coffeehouse space-cakes to Colorado dispensary exclusives such as Snoop Dogg's THC-infused gourmet chocolate bars. Prior to the legalization of recreational marijuana in California, her family owned and operated a medical marijuana collective in Shasta County. Once hemp was federally legalized, her family founded Nature's Nectar, a CBD extraction facility specializing in producing CBD Full-Spectrum Shatter sourced from organic hemp farms. In 2019 they also opened The Hive, a local CBD store in O'Fallon. She now resides in O'Fallon, Missouri, with her husband, Andrew, and daughter, McKayla.